HEART Ch

C000056364

A practical handbook for parents of children with heart conditions

Edited by Hazel Greig-Midlane
Published for Heartline Families
Charitable Incorporated Organisation
Reg no 1153442.

ISBN 978-0-9515270-4-7
© 1989, 1992, 2002, 2008, 2009, 2014, 2016 Heartline Families
1st printed September 1989
2nd Edition January 1992
3rd Edition March 2002
Amended reprint May 2008
4th edition 2009
5th edition 2016

Acknowledgements

Dr Shankhar Sridharan, Consultant Fetal and Pediatric Cardiologist, Great Ormond Street Children's Hospital, provided medical text editing, pictures and advice and a lot of his time

Sheran Taylor, for her advice on benefits

Many support groups and charities for contribution of information and graphics, in particular **Children's Heart Federation, Little Hearts Matter and Tiny Tickers**

Willow Langdale-Smith for the illustrations in *Chapter 6: Transplantation* in which she retains her copyright and intellectual property rights

John Greig-Midlane for endless proofreading, checking and wise suggestions

Dr Jasveer Mangat, Consultant Pediatric Cardiologist, for his contributions on electrophysiology.

Dr Andrew Wardle for his advice and final text editing

I thank the many contributors to earlier editions of *Heart Children:* I freely admit to having built on previous editions and updated contributions, many of which have survived from last century.

Most of all we thank the Heartline parents and children who have contributed their hard won advice and knowledge over the years to help smooth the path just a little for those who come after them; the heart children and their families whose pictures appear in these pages, and the many sponsors, without whose generosity this book could not have been published and distributed.

**This book is dedicated
to Heart Children and their Families.**

About this book

We hope this book will improve parents' knowledge and understanding. For every heart condition set out in this book there are many variations, so your child's problem may well differ from those described. Treatments are changing and improving all the time, so again your child may be offered treatment not covered here.

Heart Children is an outline and many generalisations have had to be made. What it does not do is replace the personal contact between your family and the teams involved in your child's care. Please don't be afraid to ask questions of the team looking after your child – so that you have a good understanding of the problems and plans.

We have used the terms 'heart child' and 'heart children'- this is just for convenience and to distinguish them from their brothers and sisters – they are, of course, children first and foremost, who happen to have – but are not defined by - a heart disorder.

Heartline Families publishes this book, and all profit reverts to the charity for the benefit of heart children and their families.

WARNING

This book has been prepared on the basis of information that the authors believe to be accurate. Those who are in any doubt about the medical condition of their child must consult a registered medical practitioner. The authors and publishers accept no responsibility in whatever circumstances for the actions or omissions of others occasioned by their reading this book.

COPYRIGHT

This publication is copyright. No part of this publication may be reproduced, stored in or introduced into a retrieval system in any form or by any means, or reproduced or transmitted in any form, either in part or whole, or of any nature, or be otherwise circulated in any form other than in that which it is published without the prior written permission of Heartline Families. Any person who does any unauthorised act in relation to this publication may be liable to criminal prosecution and civil claims for damages.

Introduction

As a parent when we first hear that our child has a heart problem, most of us have felt strong emotions of fear and grief.

We fear for the wellbeing of our child, for the future of our families, for the unknown and how we will deal with it. At the same time we may grieve for the loss of the normal healthy child who didn't have a heart defect, and for the pain we believe our child may suffer.

It is rare that a parent thinks a heart defect is a possibility – most of us know little about congenital heart defects, and have only heard about heart conditions in elderly people, or in those who have allowed their health to deteriorate with poor diet and lack of exercise.

Those who would normally support us – our parents and older relatives – are as likely to be as ignorant as we are initially, and to share strong emotions, which leaves them in need of support too.

Anger and guilt

Commonly we ask ourselves why this happened to our family. There is sometimes anger that other people do not seem to appreciate their healthy children, or we may feel guilty, or blame the other parent's genetic make-up for why our child is this way.

Memories of events during pregnancy can come to haunt us – the headache treated with pain killers, the night of the party, too much coffee, not enough fruit, getting pregnant at the wrong time and so on.

Whether the cause of your child's condition is found or not, anger, blame and guilt are negative emotions which we may need to work through, but quickly set aside for the good of our child, our family, ourselves.

Support

Some couples can support each other, but many find it difficult to offer support when they are dealing with their own difficult feelings. Mothers are often intimately involved with their young child – feeding or expressing breast milk, living in the hospital with a baby, dealing with the health needs and medical appointments for an older child, and may feel it easier to talk with others in a similar position.

Fathers may not be able to invest the same amount of time at a hospital. As a child's father you should expect support from friends or work colleagues. If it is not forthcoming make it clear that you have to concentrate much of your time and energy on your family, and look elsewhere for support.

In these early days, many parents have found comfort in speaking to other mothers and fathers – contacting your group, or getting involved in internet forums will often give you a circle of friends who will understand not only the emotions you feel, but also the names of defects, medical procedures, and treatments, and will sincerely sympathise with setbacks and celebrate successes.

If these are some of the problems you are dealing with, know that you will almost certainly get to the stage where you will be able to think of your child without thinking of the heart condition first, that there is every chance that this child will bring you as much joy as any other. But the effects of these emotions on you are not helpful when coming to understand your child's condition and the treatment and investigations, if any, that are needed.

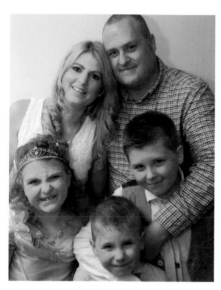

Your responsibility

You are dealing with a complex area, and your child is your responsibility – a heavy burden when decisions such as giving consent need to be made.

This book can explain some congenital heart defects and treatments, but don't be afraid to ask any question of the clinical staff, however simple you may think it.

Most children with heart problems spend most of their time with their families. It is the parents who are likely to spot problems, or can assure the doctor that their child is doing well, it is at home that medicines will be given, feeding problems solved and social and educational issues dealt with.

So this book includes information about common concerns – financial, educational and social – families' experience in daily life.

Contents

1. Understanding the heart

To understand the problem your child may have, it's best to get to grips with how the normal heart works and what it needs to do. Because the way blood moves through the heart should change shortly after birth, you may need some knowledge of the (before birth) fetal circulation as well.

How the normal heart works

The heart and lungs are in the chest, protected by the breast bone, ribs and spine. The heart pumps red blood, around the body to supply the organs with oxygen and nutrition. This blood – which now looks blue - returns to the right side of the heart and is pumped under much lower pressure to the lungs. When we breathe in, oxygen from the air moves through the thin sponge like tissues of the lungs into our blood. At the same time, carbon dioxide passes from our blood into our lungs, from where we breathe it out.

The heart is a muscle with four hollow chambers, two on the left and two on the right divided by a wall. These are called the left and right atriums and the left and right ventricles. There are four valves which make sure that the blood moves in one direction. The pressures created by the atriums and ventricles contracting and relaxing are what opens and closes the valves.

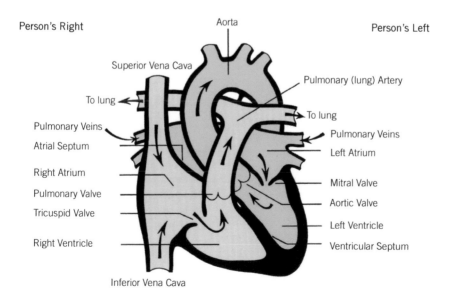

Person's Right — Aorta — Person's Left

Superior Vena Cava

Pulmonary (lung) Artery

To lung

To lung

Pulmonary Veins

Pulmonary Veins

Atrial Septum

Left Atrium

Right Atrium

Mitral Valve

Pulmonary Valve

Aortic Valve

Tricuspid Valve

Left Ventricle

Right Ventricle

Ventricular Septum

Inferior Vena Cava

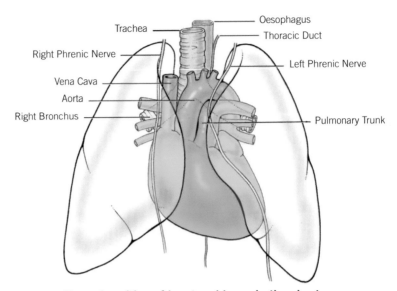

Normal position of heart and lungs in the chest

Blue blood moves towards the heart in veins which join together to become two large veins - the inferior vena cava from the lower half of the body, and the superior vena cava from the upper part of the body. This blood flows into the right atrium. the tricuspid valve opens as the atriums contract and the ventricles relax, allowing blue blood into the right ventricle. When the right ventricle contracts, blue blood is pumped through the pulmonary valve into the blood vessel called the pulmonary artery, towards the left and right lungs.

Red blood returns from the lungs in four pulmonary veins into the left atrium. When the atriums contract and the ventricles relax, the mitral valve opens, and red blood flows into the left ventricle. When the left ventricle contracts, the aortic valve opens and red blood is pumped at high pressure into the aorta. This large blood vessel divides and subdivides into all the arteries into every part of the body.

This process of contracting and relaxation, which we refer to as the heart beating, occurs between 60 and 120 beats per minute at rest.

The heart has its own complex electrical system. Its purpose is to stimulate the heart to fill with blood and to pump it rhythmically to the lungs and body. The atriums should contract at the same time to allow blood to drain through the valves into the ventricles, and then the ventricles should contract together to pump blood to the body and lungs.

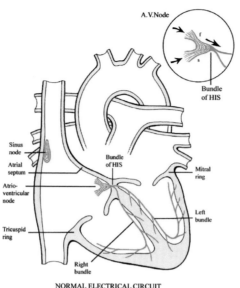

NORMAL ELECTRICAL CIRCUIT

When a child is excited or active, his or her heart should pump blood faster to provide the organs with the increased oxygen and nutrients they need, and carry away the waste, so the heart rate increases. On the other hand, when he or she is at rest you would expect the heart rate to slow down.

Before your child was born, a normal heart rate was 120-160 beats per minute – you may remember having heard the speed with which it was going during an ultrasound scan. After birth and as he or she gets older the normal rate slows down: roughly up to five months of age the resting pulse rate should be 90-140, and by the age of fifteen the normal adult pulse at rest is 60-100.

The normal heart rhythm is controlled from the sinus node, at the junction of the superior vena cava and the right atrium. This has a large supply of nerves which can speed up the heart (sympathetic) or slow it down (parasympathetic/vagus).

The electrical signal from the sinus node spreads out over the atrium causing both atriums to contract and pump blood into the ventricles. The signal then passes into the atrioventricular (a/v) node in the floor of the right atrium. There is a pause of about one to two-tenths of a second, and then the signal runs rapidly through the fast conducting system (Bundle of His) to all parts of the ventricles. This causes them to contract together, pumping blood to the lungs and the body. Then the heart muscles relax and the process starts again.

The atrium and ventricles are insulated from each other by fibrous and fatty tissue, so the only path for the electric signal should be through the Bundle of His.

The lungs are on either side of the heart and have blood vessels with thin walls to allow the exchange of carbon dioxide and oxygen. Blood pumped from the right ventricle is under low pressure, as high pressure could damage these delicate lung tissues. The left ventricle muscle is thicker and stronger than the right, as it has to pump around all parts of the body and back. The atriums' walls are thin muscle as they only have to contract to fill the ventricles.

Heart development

The heart develops from a small group of cells in the upper part of the chest of the very small embryo. These cells rapidly form a tube and the tube fold over on itself into an S shape. Bulges develop on this tube and these form the chambers of the heart and the first part of the major arteries. Between these bulges are waists. It is here that the valves develop. The heart is divided into the left and right sides by walls called septum - these grow between the two atriums, the two ventricles and also separate the big arteries – the aorta and the pulmonary artery.

By the tenth week of pregnancy the heart has connected up with the developing blood vessels in the body and the lungs. From now until the baby is born the heart and blood vessels just grow with the developing baby.

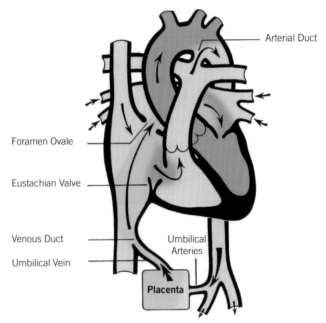

Arterial Duct

Foramen Ovale

Eustachian Valve

Venous Duct

Umbilical Vein

Umbilical Arteries

Placenta

Circulation before birth

As the baby cannot breathe until he or she is born, the lungs just have a small blood supply to allow them to grow. Before birth it is the placenta, not the lungs, which supplies the baby with oxygen and nutrition and removes carbon dioxide.

Oxygenated blood from the placenta returns to the inferior vena cava, passes through a valve into the right atrium and then through a small hole (foramen ovale) into the left atrium. From here it travels into the left ventricle and is pumped into the aorta and up to the brain. The heart muscle itself is supplied by the coronary arteries which are the first to branch from the bottom of the aorta.

The deoxygenated (blue) blood passes through the pulmonary artery through the ductus arteriosus into the descending aorta and is carried back to the placenta.

The deoxygenated blood from the top half of the body is directed to the right ventricle which pumps it into the pulmonary artery. The majority of the blood then goes into a tube – the ductus arteriosus - between pulmonary artery and the aorta, and down the aorta into the abdomen to pick up fresh oxygen from the placenta.

It is because the circulation is different before birth that the majority of babies with heart defects, even those with very severe heart problems, grow normally in the womb.

Changes after birth

The blood supply from the placenta is removed from the baby's circulation as soon as the umbilical cord is clamped. As the baby's lungs expand with crying, blood passes into them in increasing amounts.

The blood picks up the oxygen from the air, and the increased amount of blood returning to the left atrium closes the foramen ovale – the hole between the two atriums.

Over the next few days the ductus arteriosus between the pulmonary artery and the aorta closes. These changes result in an increased amount of oxygen being available to the child as a result of the lungs working. The blood pressure in the body increases and gradually, the pressure in the lungs and in the right ventricle falls.

Some heart problems may start to affect the baby as these changes in the circulation occur.

2. Prenatal diagnosis

During pregnancy most expectant mothers have an ultrasound scan. Sometimes a heart defect can be picked up or suspected by the sonographer (the person who does the scan). If this happens the expectant mother will be referred to a specialist – usually a fetal cardiologist – to get a more accurate diagnosis.

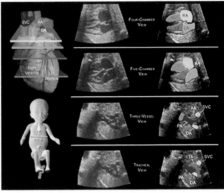

The chance of a heart problem arising again is a little higher if you already have a child with a heart defect, but it won't necessarily be the same defect. You can ask for a more detailed scan of the heart during your next pregnancy.

Reproduced by kind permission of Greggory R DeVore MD

Speak to the person arranging your maternity care – GP, midwife or local hospital – or to your child's cardiologist. This scan may be arranged early, although you may be referred after eighteen weeks when most of the structures of the heart can be seen more clearly.

Diagnosis

Even a specialist scan cannot always tell how severe a defect will be when the baby is born. Some defects improve as the fetus grows, others grow more severe. Sometimes a heart which is very abnormal – for example on the wrong side of the body - works extremely well.

A heart defect can be one of a number of symptoms of a syndrome – such as DiGeorge or Downs - so you may be offered further tests to diagnose any other condition.

Most fetal heart problems cannot be treated until the baby is born, although a very fast heart beat can sometimes be controlled by giving medicine to the mother. Some heart conditions will need to be treated as soon as the baby is born, so you will be able to make arrangements to deliver your baby safely near a hospital that can carry out children's heart surgery and catheter treatments.

The sonographer will look to see if the heart has four chambers, and if the main blood vessels, the aorta and pulmonary artery, can be seen arising. Remember that at the first scan your baby's heart is very small, no larger than a pea, and even quite big defects can be missed.

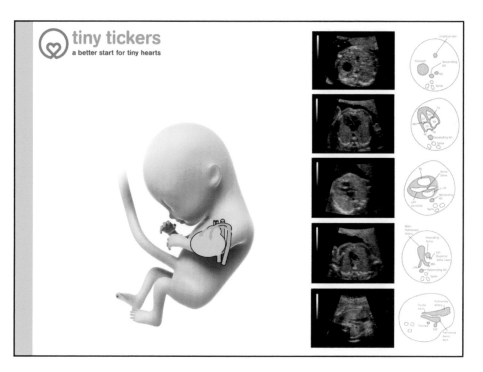

Other defects may develop late in pregnancy, or are normal features of the circulation before birth that fail to change as they should during the first few days of the baby's life.

The fetal cardiologist will be able to tell you about the kind of problems your child could have with the suspected heart defect, and how it could affect his or her life – a prognosis. At this point it can sometimes be difficult to accurately predict prognosis, including the potential for treatment. But even some very complex defects can now be treated so that the child can lead a relatively normal life, although a number of operations may be needed, including perhaps a transplant, and life expectancy may still be shortened. Other heart problems can be dealt with by non-surgical methods, some by just a single surgery. And some heart conditions may need to be monitored, but never need treatment.

Help, support and Information

See **Chapter 4** for the type of defect that could be diagnosed, **Chapter 5** for the treatment– and **Chapter 13 Sources of help and support** for a list of groups, many of which offer contact with families that have had a prenatal diagnosis of a heart defect.

Children's Heart Federation can direct you to a heart group with particular knowledge of the type of heart defect diagnosed and information about where treatment is available.

Tiny Tickers offer advice on what to ask at 20 week scan:

e: info@tinytickers.org
w: www.tinytickers.org

ARC: Antenatal Results and Choices: offers non-directive support and information to parents having to make difficult decisions about continuing or ending a pregnancy:

t: 0845 077 2290 or 0207 713 7486 from a mobile.
w: www.arc-uk.org

SANDS: stillbirth and neonatal death charity: supporting anyone affected by the stillbirth or death of a baby in the first few weeks of life.

t: 02074365881
e: helpline@uk-sands.org
w: www.uk-sands.org

Preparing for the birth

If your child needs treatment soon after he or she is born, you will need to arrange to give birth near the specialist heart hospital. Some of these hospitals have a maternity unit – this may be important to you if you are likely to have a caesarean, or more than one baby for example, and so would find travelling difficult. There may be antenatal classes especially for those expecting a child with a heart problem. Ask what accommodation there is for new mothers and fathers – talk to your GP, midwife or hospital providing your antenatal care.

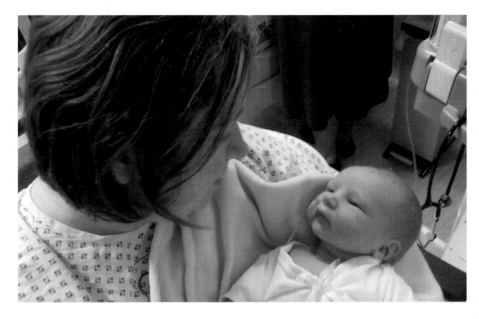

3. Diagnosing your child

If a heart condition is suspected, by a midwife, health visitor or GP, your child will probably be seen first by the pediatrician – a children's doctor – who will refer him or her on to a pediatric cardiologist – a children's heart doctor.

Heart diseases in children

Acquired heart disease

Kawasaki disease is an illness that can result in weak spots in the heart's coronary arteries. If it is treated in its early stages, there is much less chance of this happening. The cause of Kawasaki disease is not known. The symptoms are: rash, fever and peeling skin on the hands and feet.

Rheumatic fever is an inflammatory disease caused by a bacterial infection. Symptoms a week or two after a sore throat are fever and swollen joints. Damage to the heart, which mainly affects the valves, causes tiredness, breathlessness and weight loss.

Some forms of cardiomyopathy (heart muscle disease) are inherited, and some may be present at birth (ie congenital) but others seem to be acquired as a result of a viral infection. The most noticeable symptoms in children are usually breathlessness, poor feeding and fatigue after a viral illness.

Infective endocarditis is a heart condition caused by bacterial, viral and fungal infections getting into the blood stream and growing on parts of the heart. An affected child will have flu-like symptoms, with a high temperature which swings up and down over a few weeks with night sweats, fatigue and poor appetite.

Congenital heart disease

Increasingly heart defects are picked up before a baby is born - see **Chapter 2**, but the first sign of the problem may become apparent in the first few hours after birth, in the first few days or weeks of life, or sometimes not for months or even years. Many hospitals will use pulse oxymmetry at birth to check the amount of oxygen in your child's blood - saturation or 'sats'. If this is low it could be caused by a heart problem or an infection so further tests would be carried out. Shortly after your child is born, he or she will be seen by a pediatrician, who will check the baby's heart. Descriptions of the more common types of congenital defect are in **Chapter 4**.

Heart Arrhythmia

Some children experience heart rhythms that are irregular, too fast, or too slow - these may be acquired or result from congenital or inherited conditions - see **Chapters 4 and 5** for types of arrhythmia and treatments.

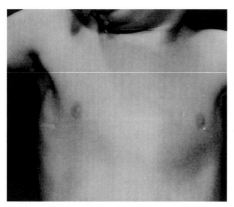

Abnormally shaped chest   **Clubbing of toes**

Diagnosis

What the doctor will look for

A baby or child who seems unwell at home may be referred to a pediatrician or GP to check his or her heart. When looking to see if a heart condition exists, the doctor will ask questions concerning your child compared to others of the same age – for example the feeding pattern of babies, sleeping pattern in the daytime of toddlers, physical activity of children at play and at school and whether there are any activities that bring on symptoms such as breathlessness or tiredness.

The doctor who examines your child will look at height and weight, as a child with a heart condition will often be small for their age. The colour of lips, tongue, fingers and toes will be checked as these can look blue (cyanosed) in some heart conditions. Nails may be misshapen (clubbing) – a sign of poor circulation.

Other tests could be

- checking the oxygen levels in the blood (oxygen saturation or sats).

- checking the pulse rate – which could be too fast or slow, weak or irregular - in the arms and legs as well as neck.

- measure blood pressure – too high or too low.

- feel the abdomen to check the size of the liver – this can become swollen in some heart conditions.

- look at the shape of the chest – this can look lopsided if the heart muscle is larger than it should be.

- listen with a stethoscope to heart sounds – the sounds produced as valves close, and murmurs – the sound of blood moving through the heart and large blood vessels.

Symptoms

These are the symptoms that the doctor will ask about and look for when first making a diagnosis, or when periodically checking a child with a heart condition.

Poor weight gain

Poor or no weight gain can be a symptom of a heart condition. A baby with a heart defect may find it hard to breathe and suck at the same time, so takes in little milk at a feed. A poor circulation means that the child's digestion is inefficient at using nutrients in food. And a hard working heart needs more energy from the calories a child does manage to eat. You may hear poor weight gain referred to as 'failure to thrive'.

Sweatiness

A child with a heart condition often sweats more than others as the system is having to work hard to get enough oxygen, and get rid of fluid.

Murmurs

Murmurs are usually entirely normal – called innocent murmurs. But a murmur may sometimes be made by blood flow across holes or through abnormal valves, for example. Murmurs may be the only sign of a heart problem when they are picked up during a routine examination or a childhood illness.

Breathlessness

Children with heart problems may often become breathless more easily than other children. This occurs either because too much or too little blood is getting to their lungs.

If too much, the lungs become heavy and your child will need more effort and energy to breathe air in and out. If your child is young this can cause poor feeding because he or she cannot breathe and suck or eat at the same time. In older children breathlessness means they can exercise less (reduced exercise tolerance). If too little blood goes to the lungs, not enough oxygen is picked up to meet the needs of muscles when they exercise. This lack of oxygen causes an increase in the rate and depth of breathing.

Blueness

Healthy people can look blue around their lips and on their fingers, often a reaction to the cold. In some heart conditions, children have a blue colouring which doesn't go away and can be seen in the mouth. This is because there isn't enough oxygen in the blood. You may hear this blueness referred to as cyanosis and a child as cyanosed (pronounced sigh-an-osed).

Dizziness, fainting and spells

Dizziness or fainting (sometimes called syncope) in a child can be caused by changes in the heart rate (arrhythmia), or by obstruction of blood flowing into the pulmonary artery or the aorta (sometimes called stenosis).

Blue spells

Blue spells are caused when the blood flow into the pulmonary artery – which carries blood to the lungs – is reduced temporarily. This is caused by a spasm of the heart muscle. For a short time, the child becomes bluer and may have a funny cry as though in distress, seems to have problems breathing, and then becomes floppy and sleepy. These spells occur in particular heart conditions. You will be told if your child is likely to have a blue spell, and what to do.

Fatigue

Children who have heart problems may be tired and lack energy. Babies and toddlers may sleep for longer during the day than others of their age, and older children may not be able to keep up with normal activities at school.

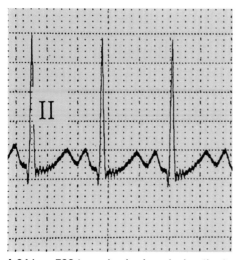

A 24 hour ECG trace showing irregular heartbeat.

Chest pain

Pain resulting from the heart condition is unusual in children. The muscles of the chest are more likely to be the source, especially if your child has had one or more operations. Children may describe the sensation of irregular heart beats as a pain in their chest.

Arrhythmia

The heart beating either too fast, too slowly, or irregularly can be a symptom of heart disease.

Fast heart beat (tachycardia: pronounced tacky-kardee-a): It is normal for your child to have a fast heart rate during and after exercise (or during and after crying in a baby), but a fast heartbeat that comes on at rest is less common and may be a symptom of a heart problem. The feeling of the heart beating heavily or quickly is called palpitations. If the fast heart beat lasts for a long time it can cause sweatiness, paleness and breathlessness. An older child may complain of a funny feeling or pain in the chest.

Slow heart beat (bradycardia: pronounced bradee-kardee-a): A heart pumping too slowly will not be able to keep an efficient circulation of the blood around the body, and this will reduce the amount of oxygen available to the organs. A child may have dizzy spells, or fainting, or complain of a feeling of discomfort in their chest or abdomen.

Fluid retention

When the heart isn't pumping well enough, it can be hard to clear fluids through the kidneys. This can result in fluid collecting in parts of the body – particularly the abdomen and liver which can become swollen. The child produces smaller amounts of urine, and may be pale, sweaty and breathless. You may notice puffiness around the eyes and swelling of the abdomen in younger children, and swollen ankles and legs in older children. Because the fluid is heavy, a child will have an unexpected sudden weight gain. This condition can be a symptom of heart failure sometimes referred to as congestive heart failure (because the fluid is causing congestion in the child's organs) – which just means that the heart is having to work much harder than normal. Until the underlying heart problem can be sorted out, fluid retention can be helped by restricting fluids or using diuretics – medicines that help the body get rid of extra fluid. **See Chapter 5 Treatments and complications.**

Tests

Not all children will need all or any of the tests here, but often tests will be needed to find the exact type of heart problem your child has and the best way of treating it. These tests may be used in diagnosing your child's condition when it is first suspected, or later to check how the heart is developing – particularly if your child has new or worsening symptoms. Some of these tests can only be carried out when your child is an inpatient. Often they will be used during an operation to help the surgeon decide on the best course of action.

If you take your child for a test such as an echo or ECG, your consent to the test doesn't have to be written down, but if the test involves sedating the child or giving an anaesthetic, or is invasive – such as a catheter test, or angiography – you will be asked to give consent after the procedure has been explained to you. You will be asked to involve your child in giving consent – to assent - so that he or she understands as far as possible what will happen and why – **see Chapter 7 Communicating, consenting, concerns and complaints.**

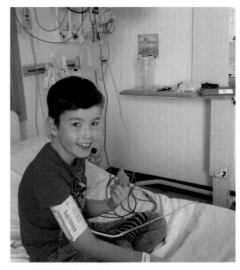

Oxygen saturation (sats)

The percentage of oxygen carried in blood compared to normal can be measured using a pulse oximeter. This is a painless, routine test.

A clip is attached to your child's finger or toe and feeds information to a monitor. A child with a heart condition will often have considerably less oxygen than the 98-100% found in the blood of a healthy child.

Oxygen saturation probe.

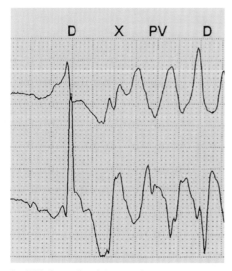

Electrocardiogram (ECG)

The ECG records the electrical impulses that come from the circuits within the heart – these will show if they are working properly, and can help in assessing if the chambers of the heart are doing extra work. While your child is awake wires are connected to sticky patches on his or her arms, legs and chest while the recording is made. The test takes about five minutes and is painless.

An ECG Recording (abnormal).

Twenty-four hour ECG

If your child has symptoms of fainting, dizziness or irregularities of the heart rhythm, he or she may need a twenty-four hour ECG, using wires attached to the chest and a small monitor that can be taken home. This can be fitted in outpatients, with your child undertaking all normal activities, other than swimming, bathing or playing in a sandpit. You may be asked to keep a record of any symptoms your child has during the time of the recording. The hospital will then play back the tape to see if any irregular heart rhythms have occurred over that period of time, and the results should come back to you via your GP or the cardiologist. This may be a different doctor, as some cardiologists are electrophysiologists, specialising in the heart's electrical circuits.

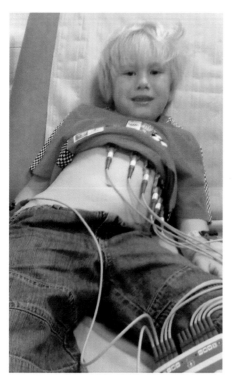

Event recorder

If your child has symptoms which could be caused by an arrhythmia, he or she can record the previous few seconds and the next few minutes of the heart's electrical activity using an event recorder. The recording can be played down a telephone or sent via the internet for analysis. If necessary this can be worn for several weeks and, if the monitor isn't waterproof, removed for bathing although increasingly waterproof devices are becoming available.

Cardiac catheter - diagnostic

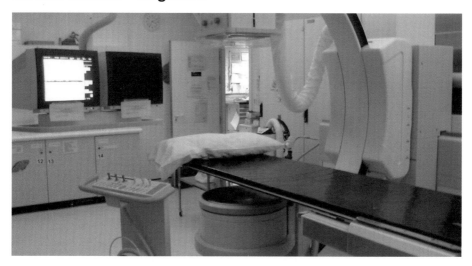

Most heart conditions can be diagnosed using echos and other tests that don't need drips or tubes inserted, but sometimes a cardiac catheterisation test is needed. Although this is not surgery it is invasive, so stringent precautions will need to be taken to prevent infection and you will not be able to stay with your child during the procedure.

A cardiac catheter is a long, fine plastic tube inserted into a vein or artery through a small puncture hole at the top of the leg or sometimes the arm or neck. The catheter can be passed into the main blood vessels and chambers of the heart and x-rays are used to help the doctor guide the catheter to the right places.

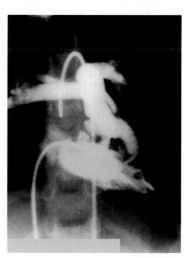

The catheter can be used to measure pressures, to take samples of blood from different parts of the heart and main blood vessels, and to inject dye into the heart (angiography) – this outlines the passage of the blood through the heart which can be seen on x-ray. This can provide useful information about the structure of the heart and can help doctors make a plan of treatment for the child.

Children who keep having fast heart beats despite treatment may need a catheter procedure to test the electrical system of the heart. The test is called an electrophysiology study. It is carried out by a cardiologist called an electrophysiologist.

The thin white lines are the catheters.

A catheter is used to steer wires into different parts of the heart to record electrical activity. Electrical impulses can be passed down the wires to try to stimulate the heart into starting and stopping the arrhythmia, so finding its source. If it can be corrected an ablation may be performed at the same time.

Tests can take several hours and are carried out under general anaesthetic in an area of the hospital reserved for carrying out catheter procedures – usually called the Cath Lab.

On return to the ward your child will be sleepy and need to rest. There may be a bruise where the catheter was inserted – usually at the top of the thigh – but you can expect to go home later that day or the following day, unless your child is being treated as an inpatient for other problems at the time.

Echocardiography (echo)

Using the sound waves from an echo machine, a good picture of the heart and its function can be seen on a screen and recorded. The pressure of blood through the valves can be measured, and direction of the blood flow shows as different colours. This scan is similar to the one used in pregnancy: a painless test, using a probe across the skin of the chest and neck. Restless younger children may need to be sedated.

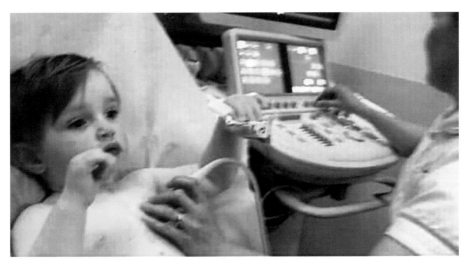

Having an echo scan

Transoesophageal Echocardiography (TOE)

This is an echo which looks at the back of the heart through the oesophagus (the tube that food goes down into the stomach) pronounced ee-soff-a-gus. It is often used for adolescents and young adults when the usual echo pictures may not be so clear. It is sometimes used to give the surgeon a clearer picture of valve function, holes in the walls between the left and right atrium, and abnormal flow in veins which bring blood back to the heart from the lungs. It will normally be done when your child is under an anesthetic as part of another procedure.

Chest x-ray

A chest x-ray can show the size and position of the heart, and which part is enlarged. It can help the doctor work out how blood is flowing through the lungs. Before an outpatient appointment you may want to check to see if your child will be having an x-ray. If there is any chance that you are pregnant, you will not be able to stay with your child so you may want to take someone else with you to stay with him or her.

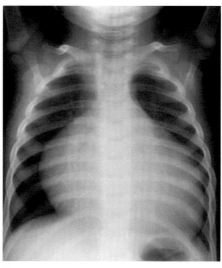

Above: a chest x-ray showing an enlarged heart.

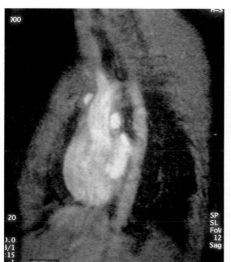
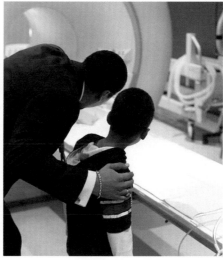

Above: a magnetic resonance image of the side of the chest, and the MRI scanner – the patient slides inside the machine. MRI enables the structures of the heart to be examined in remarkable detail. There is no discomfort except your child has to lie very still, and there is a loud buzzing noise.

Computerised Tomography Scan (CT Scan)

A CT Scan may be needed if your child is not a suitable candidate for an MRI. It is much quicker and gives good 3D pictures of the heart, but needs a small dose of radiation.

Magnetic Resonance Imaging (MRI)

MRI technology uses the body's magnetic field and high-tech computers to construct images of the heart, blood vessels, lungs and trachea. MRI can be used in virtually all patients, unless metal structures are in the chest, although some recently developed pacemakers are safe.

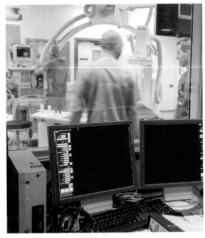

Above: CT scanning room

Radio-isotope scanning

This test can be done as an outpatient. It is used to assess the heart muscle and the amount of blood getting to the lungs. Your child will have an injection, after which he or she will need to lie still on a table for a few minutes while being scanned. Restless younger children may need to be sedated. You may be able to stay with your child during this procedure.

Barium swallow

With heart defects children sometimes have other problems, such as a narrowing of the oesophagus (food pipe) or trachea (wind pipe). If your child is suspected of having such a problem he or she may be given a thick liquid to drink, containing barium. This will show up any narrowing on x-ray. If there is any chance that you are pregnant, you will not be able to stay with your child so you may want to take someone else with you to stay with him or her.

Hemoglobin (Hb) blood test

Hemoglobin (pronounced hee-mow-glow-bin) is the chemical in the red blood cells that carries oxygen and carbon dioxide around the body. The amount of Hb in the blood may need to be measured using a blood test to make sure the level is correct. If your child is blue, he or she probably has more Hb than usual in the blood, which is an advantage, but if this is too high the blood becomes very thick and sluggish. If this happens it can be a sign that surgery is needed.

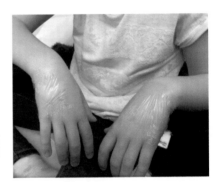

Above: magic cream

Exercise test

If your older child's exercise tolerance needs to be checked, this is usually carried out by getting him or her to walk or run on a treadmill, while recording the ECG and blood pressure. The test is particularly useful in assessing heart muscle function and heart rhythm problems.

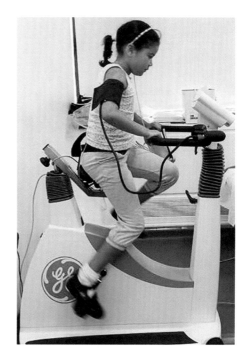

Genetic testing

Genetic testing involves taking a blood sample to see if a chromosomal problem or a genetic problem can be found. You may be offered this for your child if there is a possibility of such a result, and it will be explained fully to you.

A positive result could help alert you to other health problems. If the condition may be hereditary, then a test could help you to decide about future pregnancies, or to be aware that you yourself or other members of your family may have inherited some of the characteristics of a syndrome. Most genetic tests will not be able to tell you the reason for your child's heart condition, but this is a developing field and better tests may be available shortly.

Unique is an organisation which helps families whose child has a chromosomal problem, and there are support groups for some types of genetic defect - **see Chapter 13 Sources of help and support.**

Prognosis

The point of tests is to establish what help your child may need in the form of treatment, and what the outcome is likely to be. It may be difficult for a pediatric cardiologist (children's heart doctor) to tell you that your child will be completely well, because even the most straightforward heart conditions are different from each other. There are new treatments for the most complex conditions which seem very successful, but we need time before we can know how well children will be as adults.

Doesn't need treatment

Your child's heart defect may be of the kind that is expected to sort itself out as your child grows, and is unlikely to need treatment at any time in their life. Your child may be monitored by a local pediatrician every year or so until the problem has disappeared.

Probably won't need treatment

The condition is unlikely to affect your child in any way, and the very low risk of treating it is higher than the risk of leaving it alone.

Can be corrected with a low risk of complications

Your child may need a procedure such as closure of a duct by catheter, or surgical repair of a defect in a septum, which should result in him or her being completely well and after a routine follow-up should not need further appointments.

Can be corrected but there may be a need for treatment later

Conditions such as Fallot's Tetralogy, or Atrio-Ventricular Septal Defect can often be corrected fully, but because these conditions are variable, your child may need further treatment. A more accurate prognosis can be given to you when the defect is first repaired.

Most of the problems that arise from the heart defect can be dealt with so that your child can expect to live a normal life.

Can be palliated (improved or stopped from deteriorating) but cannot be corrected

Some hearts do not have the potential for a normal circulation. Depending on the complexity of your child's heart, surgery could provide him or her with a life that includes physical exercise, education and employment.

May need transplant

If your child has a condition that can no longer be helped with surgery or improved with medication, he or she may be assessed for a transplant – but this may be many years from the first diagnosis.

Your child's heart diagnosis

You may find it helpful to ask your consultant to use the diagrams at the back of this book to explain your child's heart condition. There are three – use one to understand the diagnosis, and the second to see what the heart looks like after treatment. There is a labelled diagram of a heart to help you compare your child's heart to a normal one.

4. Heart Problems

This chapter describes the most common heart conditions in children in alphabetical order. Your child's problem may be described here, or only partly described, or not covered at all. Have a look in the index if you can't see it – it may be called a different name.

Ask your cardiologist to use the diagram of a heart at the end of this book to show how your child's heart is affected.

For details about different kinds of treatment – catheter procedures, open and closed heart surgeries, devices and medicines – see Chapter 5.

Anomalous Pulmonary Venous Connection

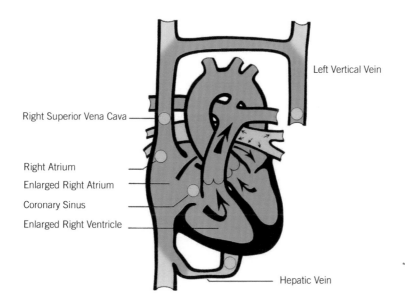

Left Vertical Vein

Right Superior Vena Cava

Right Atrium

Enlarged Right Atrium

Coronary Sinus

Enlarged Right Ventricle

Hepatic Vein

In Anomalous Pulmonary Venous Connection (APVC) pulmonary veins, which should bring red oxygenated blood from the lungs to the left side of the heart, connect to the right side of the heart instead. The diagram shows that the pulmonary veins drain into the right side of the heart instead of the left, the left vertical vein and the hepatic vein. A hole between the two sides (ASD) allows some oxygenated blood to get to the left side. Sometimes not all the pulmonary veins are involved, in which case it is called partial – PAPVC. Otherwise it is total – TAPVC.

In the right side of the heart, the oxygenated blood mixes with blue deoxygenated blood, some of which is pumped from the right atrium into the left atrium, allowing some oxygenated blood to reach the body.

If your child has the total form of this defect, he or she may be blue, breathless and struggling very early on. Once it is diagnosed, your child will need open heart surgery as soon as possible to reconnect the pulmonary veins into the left side of the heart.

The partial form of the defect will also need surgery, but there may be a period when your child is stabilised and allowed to grow – the larger the heart, the easier it is for the surgeon to operate successfully.

Long term follow up will be needed as the pulmonary veins sometimes narrow and restrict blood flow as the child grows, and an irregular heartbeat can develop after surgery.

Atrial Septal Defect

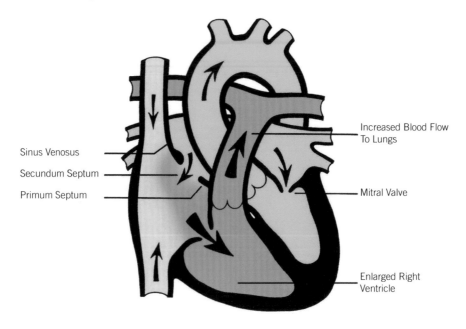

An Atrial Septal Defect (ASD) is a hole between the left and right atriums.

Before a baby is born his or her circulation depends on a flap valve – a one way route – between the atriums, called the foramen ovale. In most cases, this closes shortly after birth. If it does not, some oxygenated blood will be forced by the higher pressure in the left atrium into the right atrium. A foramen ovale which does not close is called a Patent Foramen Ovale – or PFO. Sometimes the PFO is so big that the large amount of blood shunted from the left to the right side of the heart, and pumped into the lungs, makes the baby breathless, and in need of treatment.

A hole in the lower part of the atrial septum – the wall between the atriums – is called a Primum Defect. It may be associated with an abnormality of the mitral valve, causing it to leak. You may hear the name Sinus Venosus used to describe a hole near the top of the atrial septum. This can be associated with a defect of a vein bringing blood back to the heart from the right lung – the right pulmonary vein, a form of PAPVC.

Sometimes a child will have symptoms - frequent chest infections and problems putting on weight – but an ASD may not be found in a young child who has no symptoms, until a heart murmur is picked up at a routine examination.

Small ASDs that allow little blood to shunt from one side of the heart to the other do not cause problems and will sometimes close by themselves.

Those which are larger cause the heart to work harder and to start failing in adulthood, and the fragile arteries in the lungs may be damaged by the extra blood being pumped into them.

Some ASDs can be closed without needing surgery. Instead, a catheter is threaded through a vein into the heart and the ASD is sealed using a device that stays in place when the catheter is withdrawn. This procedure leaves no permanent scarring, and needs a very short hospital stay – one or two days - if your child is otherwise well.

Your child may have an ASD with a number of other defects – and in some cases ASDs are created to increase the amount of blood getting to a child's lungs. These may be dealt with when other corrective surgery is carried out.

Those defects which cannot be closed by catheter method may need open heart surgery so that the surgeon can get to the site of the ASD and close it safely, while repairing any other structures of the heart associated with the defect.

Aortic Stenosis

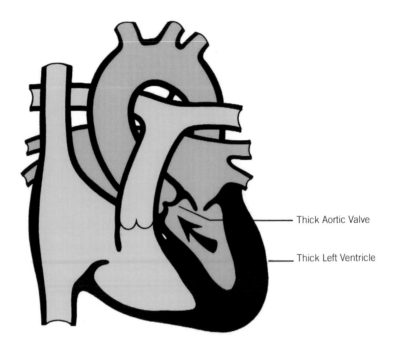

Thick Aortic Valve

Thick Left Ventricle

Aortic Stenosis (AS) is a narrowing between the left ventricle and the aorta – a part of the heart which may be referred to as the left ventricular outflow tract (LVOT).

Your child may not show any signs of having this condition, even if the blood flow is severely restricted. Symptoms can be breathlessness and fainting.

Older children with moderate to severe obstruction should avoid competitive sport, rowing, judo and karate while awaiting treatment. Once your child is diagnosed, and as long as immediate treatment is not needed, a check will be kept on how hard the left ventricle has to work to get blood through the narrowing (stenosis). This may be by echocardiogram – a scan over the chest – and sometimes transoesophageal echo (TOE) is used. In this case, your child will be sedated under anaesthetic and the echo carried out by inserting a tube into the oesophagus from where a better view of the root of the aorta can be seen.

The most common form is **Aortic Valve Stenosis** – the leaflets of the aortic valve are thick, and restrict the amount of oxygenated blood pumped from the left ventricle into the aorta. The valve may be bicuspid – that is it has two instead of three leaflets or cusps.

Using a catheter threaded through the blood vessel in the groin, to the heart and into the aorta, a balloon can be inflated and pulled through to increase the size of the opening to the aorta. This technique – dilatation, valvoplasty or balloon stretching – is safe and effective, but can result in leaking through the valve, and may have to be repeated more than once while waiting for corrective surgery.

Sometimes surgery is the first option considered, or may be offered after balloon stretching – surgery needs the heart to be stopped and opened. The surgeon may be able to stretch the valve or free it to move more efficiently, but often it will need to be replaced. The valve is removed and an artificial valve is sewn into its place. Although artificial valves are very effective, your child may have to take blood thinning medicine (anticoagulants) which could limit his or her activities because of the risk of bruising and need regular blood tests. Also artificial valves cannot grow with the child, so if he or she is small, a replacement may be needed within a few years.

The alternative to an artificial valve is to use your child's own pulmonary valve as a replacement for the aortic valve. This is called the Ross Procedure: the advantages are that the valve will grow with your child, and anticoagulants will not be needed. The pulmonary valve is then replaced, and if it fails in the future, your child may be offered the technique for replacing it using a catheter procedure rather than surgery.

Your child's new aortic valve may be referred to as an autograft (from within the same person) and the new pulmonary valve as a homograft – a valve donated by another person.

With **Subaortic Stenosis**, a shelf of muscle grows between the left ventricle and the aortic valve, partially blocking blood pumped into the aorta. In some cases the blockage is caused by thin tissue growing across the aortic valve. In either case, when the obstruction is severe open heart surgery will be needed to remove it. On most occasions, surgical removal of the obstruction is successful. Occasionally, the removal of muscle may need a Konno Procedure (see page 74) which may be combined with replacement of the aortic valve. This is needed when the outflow tract is too small for the child's size.

With **Supra Aortic Stenosis** there is a narrowing in the aorta above the aortic valve. If the obstruction is severe, the aorta will need to be patched, using open heart surgery.

Your child will need long-term follow-up after any of these treatments.

Atrial Isomerism

Your child's condition may be described to you as Right Atrial Isomerism or Left Atrial Isomerism. If he or she has the Right Isomerism (sometimes referred to as Asplenia Syndrome, or Ivemark Syndrome) the upper two chamber of the heart look like right atriums, whereas in the Left Isomerism (sometimes called Polyspenia) there are two left type of atriums. As a result the heart defects are often very severe and complex. In Right Isomerism these often include Atrio-Ventricular Septal Defect, Transposition of the Great Arteries, Pulmonary Stenosis or Atresia and Anomalous Pulmonary Venous

Connection. Your child will have no spleen, which leaves him or her susceptible to infection.

If your child has Left Atrial Isomerism the most likely defects are Atrio-Ventricular Septal Defect, a slow heart beat (Bradycardia) due to Complete Heart Block. He or she may have several small spleens, although this may not cause any health problem.For both Left and Right Atrial Isomerism, there is a chance of the bowel twisting due to an associated abnormal folding.

Atrio-Ventricular Septal Defect
Complete Atrio-Ventricular Septal Defect

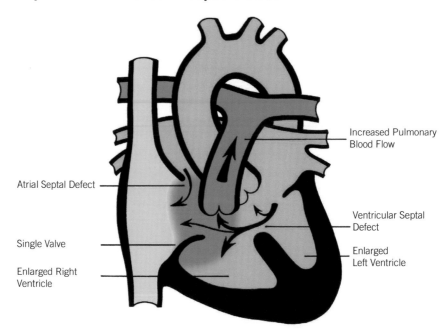

Increased Pulmonary Blood Flow

Atrial Septal Defect

Ventricular Septal Defect

Single Valve

Enlarged Left Ventricle

Enlarged Right Ventricle

In complete Atrio-Ventricular Septal Defect (CAVSD) there is a large hole in the wall between the atriums (ASD), and a large hole between the ventricles (VSD). Instead of a mitral valve and a tricuspid valve, there is only a single valve in the middle of the heart. The mitral valve is the left atrioventricular valve, and the tricuspid the right atrioventricular valve, so you may hear this single valve referred to as the atrioventricular (AV) valve.

Because pressure is higher on the left side of the heart, red oxygenated blood returning from the lungs is pumped into the right atrium through the ASD and into the right ventricle through the VSD. This excess blood is pumped by the right ventricle into the pulmonary artery and to the lungs, where the additional pressure can cause damage to the arteries. At the same time the single valve often leaks so that blood is pumped backwards from the left ventricle to the lungs. So the baby's lungs are dealing with extra blood flow making him or her breathless, and an insufficient amount of blood is getting into the aorta to take oxygen to the body to meet its needs.

Your baby was probably diagnosed before or shortly after birth, as he or she would have been in trouble quite early on, being too breathless to feed and too tired to do anything but sleep. It may be suggested if the pressure is very high in your child's lungs, that a band is placed around the pulmonary artery to reduce the pressure in the lungs for a while. If your child is in heart failure, you may be asked to give him or her medicine to get rid of the excess fluid that builds up when the heart is not meeting the needs of the body. Often your child will need medicine to help the left ventricle pump efficiently.

Repair of the complete AVSD will be in early infancy. The holes are patched and the single valve is divided into two, with the middle portions of the valve attached to the patch. This surgery can completely correct the defect. Your child will need to be followed up as there is a possibility that the valves will leak, and this may increase over time, sometimes needing further surgery. You may also find that your child develops a slow heart beat (Bradycardia) which may need correcting with a pacemaker if it does not improve.

Partial Atrio-Ventricular Septal Defect

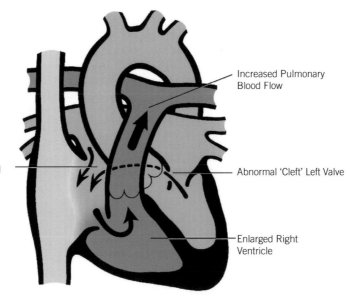

Increased Pulmonary Blood Flow

'Primum' Atrial Septal Defect

Abnormal 'Cleft' Left Valve

Enlarged Right Ventricle

33

In PAVSD there is a large hole in the wall between the two atriums (ASD) near the middle of the heart. The mitral valve (which controls blood flow on the left side of the heart) and the tricuspid valve (which controls blood flow on the right) may be leaky as a result.

Some of the red oxygenated blood from the higher pressure left atrium will be pumped into the right atrium, through the tricuspid valve into the right ventricle, and from here through the pulmonary valve and into the lungs. Your child may not have been diagnosed as a young baby as he or she may have been able to cope with the defect quite well, and it did not interfere with the activities of breathing, eating, and growing. The murmur of extra blood passing through the valves may have been heard when your child was examined by the GP.

Over time, your child's lungs may be damaged by the pressure of the extra blood being pumped to them, and the valves may become more leaky and inefficient, so treatment will be needed before these occur. PAVSD will need open heart surgery, during which the hole is patched and the valve or valves repaired with a stitch. Your child will need long term follow-up to make sure the valves are working properly.

Bradycardia

Bradycardia (pronounced brad-ee-card-ee-a) means that the heart rate is too slow. Your child may not have any symptoms, and it was discovered when his or her pulse was checked for some other reason, or there may have been dizziness, tiredness and breathlessness.

The problem may be that the heart's natural pacemaker - the sinus node - is too slow, or that there is a problem within the atrioventricular node. When there is some reason why signals cannot pass normally from the atrium to the ventricles, the ventricles depend on generating their own pacing, and tend to contract at too slow a rate to meet the body's demands – this condition is called heart block.

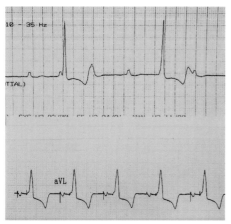

Upper trace 1: Complete heart block (slow ventricular rate).

Lower trace 2: Pacing spikes from implanted pacemaker precede atrial and ventricular signals.

The reasons for your child's bradycardia can normally be established using an ECG. Sometimes he or she will need to have a 24-hour ECG. This can be carried out at home after the tape is put on in the hospital. Stickers are attached to the chest and if your son or daughter is old enough, the recording device can be carried comfortably during normal activities at home or at school. Of course, swimming and bathing will not be possible while the recorder is in place.

A stress test may occasionally be needed: this is an ECG recording while your child exercises on a treadmill or a stationary bike.

Some cases of Heart Block – after surgery for example – will resolve as the heart recovers from the trauma of the operation, and so your child may need several examinations to confirm whether treatment is needed or not.

Treatment for Complete Heart Block may not be needed unless the heart rate is very low or your child has symptoms such as dizziness or breathlessness. Treatment is normally by using a pacemaker. The pacemaker box is inserted under the skin near the armpit, and one or two leads are attached to the heart. Although this may be done during the course of a bigger open heart surgery, it is usually carried out in the catheter laboratory.

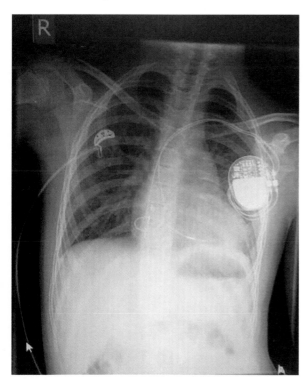

Above: Pacemaker in place

Replacement of the battery part of the pacemaker in older children can be carried out under a local anaesthetic. Pacemakers can be put into newborns – obviously very important if your baby was diagnosed before birth – and the leads or battery parts need to be replaced as your child uses up the battery and as he or she grows. Checks to find out how well the pacemaker is working, how much battery is left and changing the programme so that the pacing speeds up or slows done, are carried out by sending electric signals from outside the chest. This is not a painful procedure, takes only a few minutes and can be done at an outpatient appointment.

Coarctation of the Aorta

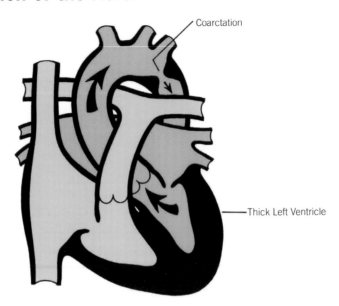

Coarctation

Thick Left Ventricle

Coarctation means a narrowing. Coarctation of the Aorta (COA) is a narrowing in the aorta, the main artery carrying oxygenated blood from your child's heart to the body. The narrowing in the aorta means that the left ventricle which pumps red oxygenated blood into the aorta – is having to work much harder. As a consequence of the coarctation, the blood pressure is increased in the top of the body, and reduced in the lower half and the legs.

If your baby's narrowing is very severe, he or she may be breathless, have difficulties in feeding, and may become more unwell. A moderate narrowing may not have been found until your child was older. A murmur – produced by the sound of blood going through the aortic valve – may be heard when your child is examined by a doctor, and the pulses in his or her legs are found to be weak.

If your child has high blood pressure or other symptoms, the narrowing will need to be removed. If there is only a mild obstruction, your child will be reviewed regularly in outpatients to check that the narrowing is not getting worse.

Some narrowings can be dealt with by ballooning – instead of surgery, a catheter is threaded through the artery or vein in the groin to the position of the narrowing, and a balloon is inflated to stretch the aorta. In older children, a stent, a mesh tube, can be inserted and left in place. This holds the aorta open.

If surgery is needed, the operation is carried out through the left side of the chest or through the breastbone. The heart does not need to be stopped, so the heart-lung machine is not used. The narrow section is removed, or patched with artificial material. Sometimes the first part of the artery to the left arm can be used to repair it.

Recovery is usually straightforward. Long term follow up will be needed to check your child's blood pressure for any evidence of recurrence of the narrowing - more likely to occur if the operation is performed during the first few months of life. If this happens, balloon stretching of the narrow area with a catheter or further surgery may be necessary.

Dilated Cardiomyopathy

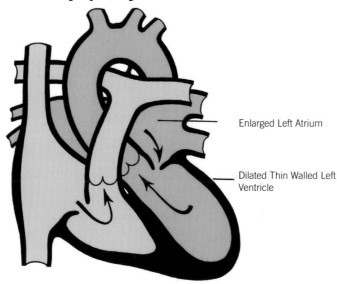

Enlarged Left Atrium

Dilated Thin Walled Left Ventricle

Dilated Cardiomyopathy (DCM) can affect your child at any age.

The heart muscle cannot pump blood properly, as it is thin and baggy. This leaves the lungs full of fluid and the body short of oxygen. As a result, your child may become breathless, have problems with feeding (particularly if he or she is very young), and with tiredness and exhaustion after physical activity.

DCM is an umbrella term describing an abnormal heart muscle, and there could be many causes - such as inherited condition, or infection. Diuretics are used to allow your child's body to get rid of excess fluid, and anticoagulants will help to prevent blood clots forming in the sluggish flow within the heart. Your child may recover completely, but if the condition does not respond to medication and worsens, he or she may be assessed for a heart transplant. If your child becomes much worse, bridging treatment in the form of a Ventricular Assist Device (VAD) may be offered, whilst waiting for a new heart to become available. A VAD is implanted surgically and acts as a pumping mechanism for the heart.

Double Inlet Ventricle

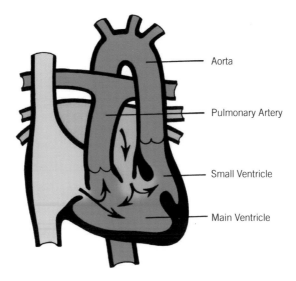

- Aorta
- Pulmonary Artery
- Small Ventricle
- Main Ventricle

This defect may have been described to you as Double Inlet Left Ventricle (DILV) or Double Inlet Right Ventricle (DIRV), which is shown in the diagram above. If your child has been found to have either of these, he or she will have just one ventricle receiving blue deoxygenated blood and red oxygenated blood. Although only a single ventricle is pumping blood to both the body and the lungs, there is usually a second, smaller, ventricle alongside. There may be only one valve (the atrioventricular or a/v valve) between the atriums and the ventricles, instead of two.

Sometimes the pulmonary artery and aorta both arise from the large ventricle, so that mixed red and blue blood is pumped directly to the lungs and to the body. It is more usual to find the arteries arising one from each ventricle, with a hole between the two ventricles (VSD) so that some red and blue blood is pumped through into the smaller ventricle.

Your child's pulmonary artery may have high pressure, unless there is a narrowing or obstruction to it, in which case insufficient blood will be getting to the lungs. As you can tell, this is a very variable condition and your child will need to be assessed to see what treatment will be needed in his or her case.

If he or she is blue and breathless, there may be a need to connect more blood into the lungs by using a shunt from the aorta to pulmonary artery, or using a catheter to stretch the narrowing. If there is too much pressure in the lungs, there may be a need for the main pulmonary artery to be banded, so that the lungs are protected.

If there is narrowing between the main ventricle and the aorta, or actually in the aorta, then this will need to be relieved, so that sufficient oxygenated blood can be pumped to the body.

Planned treatment for your child may involve two or three operations, which will eventually allow blue deoxygenated blood coming back from the body to be connected directly into the pulmonary artery. This separates the blue deoxygenated blood from the red oxygenated blood, and allows the pumping power of the ventricle to move blood around the body and back to the heart.

Long-term follow-up is needed to check your child's arteries and heart rhythm.

Ebstein's Anomaly

Courtesy of Children's Heart Federation

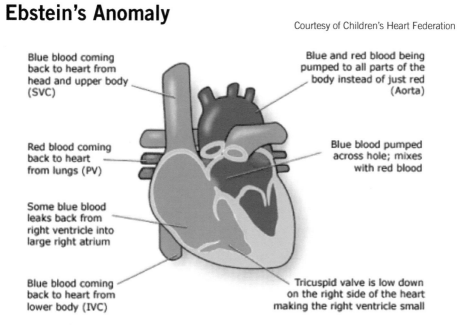

Blue blood coming back to heart from head and upper body (SVC)

Blue and red blood being pumped to all parts of the body instead of just red (Aorta)

Red blood coming back to heart from lungs (PV)

Blue blood pumped across hole; mixes with red blood

Some blue blood leaks back from right ventricle into large right atrium

Blue blood coming back to heart from lower body (IVC)

Tricuspid valve is low down on the right side of the heart making the right ventricle small

Ebstein's Anomaly is a condition, which varies from extremely serious and difficult to treat to such a mild defect that it may never be spotted in a lifetime.

The tricuspid valve, located between the right atrium and right ventricle, should prevent blue deoxygenated blood from being pumped backwards when the ventricle contracts. But in this condition, the valve is malformed, and sits well down in the ventricle. The result is that smaller amounts of blood can get into the reduced sized ventricular chamber, and some of this will leak backwards through the valve, instead of into the lungs.

There is often a hole between the right and left atrium – an Atrial Septal Defect (ASD), and your child may also suffer from attacks of a fast heart beat – a Tachycardia. If your child's symptoms are not affecting him or her, then an infrequent check will be kept on the function of the valve. If on the other hand, he or she is struggling because of shortage of blood reaching the lungs for oxygenation – blue, breathless and failing to develop normally – treatment will be needed.

Medicines can support the heart and control the fast heart beat, or the tricuspid valve can be repaired by surgery, so it no longer leaks, and the ASD can be closed. Sometimes a replacement (prosthetic) tricuspid valve may be needed
Ablation, a catheter procedure, may be offered to prevent the fast heart beat.

Fallot's Tetralogy

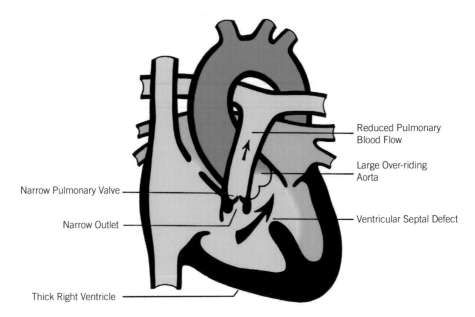

Reduced Pulmonary Blood Flow

Large Over-riding Aorta

Narrow Pulmonary Valve

Narrow Outlet

Ventricular Septal Defect

Thick Right Ventricle

Fallot's Tetralogy (FT) is sometimes referred to as Tetralogy of Fallot. (The abbreviation TOF is also used for Tracheo-Oesophageal Fistula where a baby is born with the oesophagus joined to the trachea.)

FT is a complicated defect with a hole between the two ventricles (Ventricular Septal Defect: VSD), and a narrowing between the right ventricle and the pulmonary artery (Pulmonary Stenosis: PS). The right ventricle has to work at high pressure to pump the blood through the narrowing to the lungs, so some blue deoxygenated blood is pumped through the VSD and into the aorta.

All children with FT will need surgery, although its effects can be quite mild, and not cause problems during your child's first year or so. But it can also be very severe: your baby may be too breathless to feed normally. If the baby is very blue because of narrowing extending into the pulmonary arteries, you may be offered an operation (Blalock-Taussig Shunt - BT Shunt) or a PDA stent may be a possibility (into the duct from the fetal circulation - if it is still open) or a RVOT stent across the narrow right ventricular outlet tract to increase the amount of blood to the lungs for oxygenation. The heart does not have to be stopped for this operation, but your child may have to spend time in intensive care as the body has to deal with this change in circulation. Hopefully the shunt will allow your child to grow to the point where his or her heart can be corrected more safely.

You may find that before any surgery, your child has 'spells': these are episodes when the blood flow to his or her lungs is reduced for a while. The child may cry abnormally as though in discomfort, breathe quickly, become bluer than usual, and perhaps have glazed eyes, whimper and become limp, pale and then pass off to sleep. If this should happen, hold your child over your shoulder, bringing the knees up so that they are between his or her tummy, and your chest. This will quickly improve your child's circulation and make him or her more comfortable.

Of course, you should let your child's GP and cardiologist know if this happens. There are medicines which can reduce the spells and their severity, and you will probably find that your child will be put on the list for surgery, if he or she isn't already at this point.

The surgery for FT is usually corrective – that is your child's circulation will be normal. During surgery, the heart has to be stopped and the heart- lung machine used while the VSD is patched and the narrowing across the pulmonary valve is stretched open – sometimes this may need patching as well, or a replacement valve.

The long-term results are usually very good. Sometimes in the future, a further operation may be required in those children who have a lot of blood leaking back from the pulmonary artery into the right ventricle. This is more likely if your child required a large patch across the pulmonary valve at the time of the initial operation. A new donor valve (most frequently a homograft) is inserted which improves the efficiency of the circulation and helps to reduce rhythm disturbances. The valve replacement may be by an open heart surgery or by a catheter method.

Hole in the Heart

Most of us will have heard the expression 'Hole in the Heart'. One of the most common heart conditions is a hole between the two sides of the heart. If this is between the atriums – the collecting chambers – it is called an Atrial Septal Defect: ASD - see page 28. Between the ventricles, it is called a Ventricular Septal Defect: VSD - see page 60.

There are many sizes and kinds of septal defects – they can be large or small. Generally speaking the smaller ones don't cause too much of a problem and many even close up of their own accord. But it can depend on where the hole is - it could interfere with the efficient functioning of a valve, or cause extra muscle to build blocking a pathway. Larger holes mean that too much blood passes from the high pressure left side of the heart – the left atrium or left ventricle – to the lower pressure right side – the right atrium or right ventricle.

If your baby's heart has other defects, it may be essential to keep the duct open or to create holes between the two sides of the heart. A hole is sometimes made, or deliberately left, to help the heart deal with increased pressures as a result of surgery – this is called a Fenestration.

Hypertrophic Cardiomyopathy

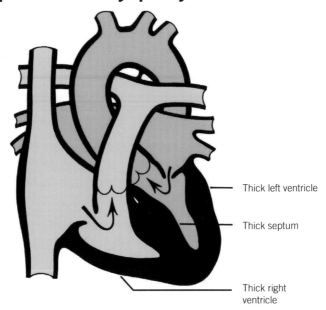

Thick left ventricle

Thick septum

Thick right ventricle

Because Hypertrophic Cardiomyopathy (HCM) is an inherited heart condition, your child may have been tested and had it discovered because of illness in a parent or sibling. Your child's case may be mild with no symptoms, or he or she may have been diagnosed because of dizziness, fainting attacks, palpitations (awareness of the heart beating) and chest discomfort.

In HCM, the heart muscle is very thick and has difficulty in relaxing. This means that less blood is pumped to your child's body and there is a shortage of oxygen as a result. Sometimes the extra muscle causes obstruction below the aortic valve, further reducing the outflow of oxygenated blood to the organs. There can be disruption in the heart's electrical circuits, causing irregular heart rates (Arrhythmia).

Medicines can improve relaxation of your child's heart, and control the heart rhythm. Surgery which may help your child includes a pacemaker to regulate a slow heart rate, an Implantable Cardioverter Defibrillator (ICD) which shocks the heart back into rhythm, and removal of the muscle obstructing the aortic valve in the area called the left ventricular outflow tract (LVOT). A catheter procedure to reduce the obstruction can be used in some children.

Your child will need advice from their Consultant or Named Nurse on what physical activities to avoid. In the longer term, if the condition cannot be stabilised your child may be assessed for a heart transplant.

Hypoplastic Left Heart Syndrome

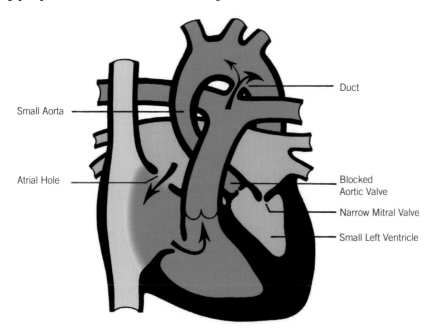

In Hypoplastic Left Heart Syndrome (HLHS), the left side of the heart and the aorta have not developed properly – the aorta is often very narrow, the aortic and mitral valve blocked or very tight and the left ventricle is small.

If your child's condition was discovered before birth, you will be advised to deliver at a time when there is a place in a specialist children's heart hospital.

Immediately after birth, your baby will be examined to find the best way of improving the amount of red oxygenated blood available to the body. At first this will have to use the fetal circulation – red blood crossing from the left to right atrium, where it mixes with blue deoxygenated blood, through the tricuspid valve and into the right ventricle. From here it will be pumped into the pulmonary artery and then to the lungs, but some will go through the ductus arteriosus.

If your child wasn't diagnosed before birth he or she would have become extremely ill, as the fetal circulation starts to close down and little oxygenated blood reaches the body. Because the left side of the heart should have the strongest pumping capacity – to get oxygenated blood all around the body and back to the heart again – this is a very difficult condition to treat.

Usually the first treatment will be to give your baby medicine to keep the PDA open - a remnant of fetal circulation within the heart. If your child is suitable, you are likely to be offered the Norwood Procedure. This involves a series of palliative operations, which gradually increases the amount of blood being pumped to the body by the right ventricle, with the aim of making this exclusively red oxygenated blood.

HLHS is a very difficult condition to treat, but your child has a better chance of surviving childhood than ever before. Successful treatment will have left him or her with a circulation dependent on the low pressure right side of the heart so it will always be abnormal and problems may arise with growth and activity. A heart transplant may be an option but because treatment has only been offered since the 1990s, there is little information about how people with HLHS cope as adults.

Long QT Syndrome

Long QT Syndrome is a fault in the heart's electrics which can result in a very fast rhythm in the ventricles (Ventricular Tachycardia) and can cause a sudden loss of heart beat. There are rarely any symptoms, although your child may have been checked for it, if he or she has had blackouts. It is more likely that your child has been examined because this condition is known to be inherited and has been diagnosed in another member of the family.

The diagnosis is made when the interval between the Q and T points on an electrocardiogram is longer than it should be. Unfortunately although your child may not have this delayed interval at the time of the recording, he or she can still have or may develop Long QT.

Once it is diagnosed, medication can prevent sudden loss of pulse, and in cases where family members are known to have died suddenly, a pacemaker or Implantable Cardioverter Defibrillator (ICD), which delivers a shock to the heart to start it again, may be considered the best treatment. There are some precautions that your child will be advised to take, including avoiding strenuous sports and some medicines.

Persistent Arterial Duct or Patent Ductus Arteriosus (PDA)

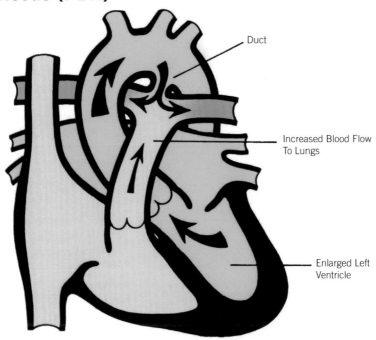

Duct

Increased Blood Flow
To Lungs

Enlarged Left
Ventricle

Patent Ductus Arteriosus (PDA) is sometimes known as Persistent Arterial Duct. Before birth, when the fetus was not breathing for itself – oxygen was supplied from the mother's blood through the placenta and the umbilical cord. Blood is pumped by the baby's heart, but through the right side of the heart to the left, bypassing the lungs, and into the aorta, through an artery called the ductus arteriosus.

As the baby takes its first breaths, the fetal circulation disappears and starts to close the ductus. If the ductus arteriosus doesn't close (is persistent), some of the red blood being pumped to the body at high pressure is forced into the lower pressure pulmonary artery via this duct, and into the lungs.

If your baby's heart has other defects, it may be essential to keep the duct open. Otherwise if only a small amount is escaping, there may be no problem, but if the duct is still open (patent) after three months it is unlikely to close on its own. A large duct in a small baby, especially a premature baby, will probably need to be closed early to avoid damage to the lungs and to help the baby grow. Your child's Consultant will advise you on whether it's best to close the PDA by a catheter procedure or surgery. If a catheter procedure is best, the catheter is threaded into the vein and artery will be accessed in the same way a blood test or cannual/drip is carried out. Using dyes injected under x-ray machine visualisation (Fluoroscopy), a coil or plug is positioned and then expanded to close the duct. Any leak through the duct usually reduces and stops of its own accord. Before going home, your child will have an ECG, chest x-ray and an echocardiogram to make sure the device is in the correct position and check for a leak. The major advantages for this technique over heart surgery is that your child will have nearly no scarring and will be able to go home within a day or two of the procedure. After one or two routine checks, he or she can be discharged.

If the PDA is large and your child small, surgery is often the best solution. A small cut is made through the left side of your child's chest, through which the ductus is tied, clipped or divided. This operation does not need the heart to be stopped, so your child's recovery should be uncomplicated and without the need for intensive care. He or she will usually be sent home within two or three days with a normal heart.

Pulmonary Atresia with Intact Ventricular Septum

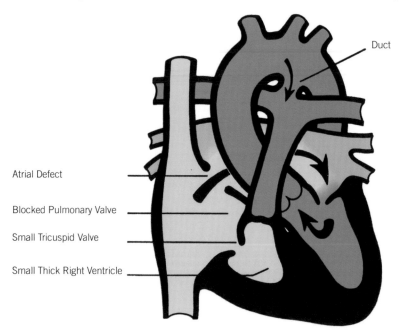

Duct

Atrial Defect

Blocked Pulmonary Valve

Small Tricuspid Valve

Small Thick Right Ventricle

Pulmonary Atresia means that the pulmonary valve, between the right ventricle and the pulmonary artery, is blocked or has never developed. Blue deoxygenated blood can only get to the lungs from the right atrium through the foramen ovale – a flap valve between the two atriums which usually closes soon after birth– then mixes with red oxygenated blood in the left atrium, through the mitral valve into the left ventricle, from where it is pumped through the aortic valve and into the aorta. From here, some blood is pumped through the ductus arteriosus – again part of your baby's circulation before birth, which normally should close soon after birth.

This condition may also be called hypoplastic right heart. Because blue blood mixes with the red blood being pumped around the body, your baby may look blue. The lack of blood flow to his or her lungs will mean that there is insufficient oxygen reaching the body for normal growth. In addition, your child may be breathless and difficult to feed.

The first steps usually taken are to keep the blood flowing to the lungs, by giving medicine to keep the duct open, and by making the hole between the atriums bigger using a balloon catheter and to stretch this.

Your baby will then have to be assessed for further treatment, which would be palliative surgery to create a single-ventricle circulation (Fontan). Sometimes, if the right ventricle isn't too small, the pulmonary valve can be opened by catheter method, stretched or even removed altogether by surgery. At the same time, an additional shunt may need to be created between the arteries carrying blood to the body, by attaching one of them to the pulmonary arteries, taking blood to the lungs. Your child will almost certainly need further surgery in the future to keep the passage into the pulmonary artery open – perhaps by inserting a tube with a valve inside it between the right ventricle and pulmonary artery, or by further balloon stretching procedures using a catheter. If your child cannot exercise and has low saturation levels of oxygen in the blood, he or she may have a Glenn Shunt: the superior vena cava, the big blood vessel bringing blue deoxygenated blood from the upper body to the heart, is attached directly to the pulmonary arteries.

This may be enough to supply the lungs, but if your child's right ventricle is never likely to grow enough to pump effectively to the lungs, operations to allow the blue deoxygenated blood to flow to the pulmonary artery - bypassing the right ventricle and pulmonary valve and sometimes the right atrium – can be carried out.

This should get your child through two or three years of normal activity. After this time, you may find your son or daughter has started to slow down, may look bluer, become breathless, and start avoiding stairs and other forms of exercise.

Further surgery can help when the blue deoxygenated blood from the lower body, carried by a blood vessel into the heart called the inferior vena cava, is connected in to the pulmonary artery – this is called the Total Cavo-Pulmonary Connection.

These Fontan-style operations to increase flow of blue blood to the lungs are being improved all the time.

During these operations any existing holes between the two sides of your child's heart will be closed, perhaps leaving a small hole between the atriums – a Fenestration – to help the heart adjust to the change in pressures less abruptly. The hole may close of its own accord, or need closing using a catheter procedure later.

After these surgeries, because the blood is flowing more slowly to the lungs as it has no pumping impetus from the right ventricle, there is a danger of blood clots forming. Your child may be given either aspirin or warfarin – both act as anticoagulants to stop this dangerous event happening.

The operations to improve (palliate) your child's condition do not correct his or her circulation, but should allow him or her to undertake most normal activities because of improved oxygen saturation.

It is not unusual for arrhythmias to occur as your child gets older, and these can be treated with medicines or by Catheter Ablation. Long term follow up should allow these to be diagnosed and treated soon after they occur.

Pulmonary Atresia with Ventricular Septal Defect

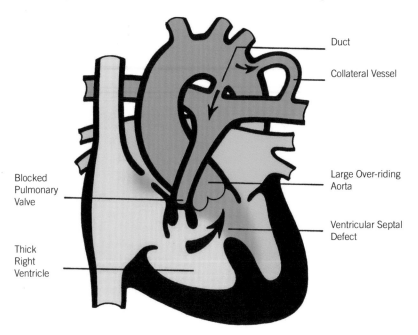

Pulmonary Atresia means that the pulmonary valve, between the right ventricle and the pulmonary artery, is blocked or has never developed. A Ventricular Septal Defect is a hole between the two ventricles.

Blue deoxygenated blood can only reach the lungs from the right ventricle by passing through the hole (VSD) into the left ventricle and then mixing with red oxygenated blood as it is pumped into the aorta. From here some may be pumped through the ductus arteriosus – if it is open – it is part of your baby's circulation before birth which should close soon afterwards.

Often there are a number of small arteries from the aorta to the pulmonary artery (Major Aorto-Pulmonary Collateral Arteries known as MAPCAs) which carry blood to one or both lungs. Because blue blood mixes with red, your baby may look blue. The lack of blood flow to his or her lungs may mean that there is insufficient oxygen reaching the body for normal growth. Your child may be breathless and difficult to feed. Too many MAPCAs may create the same effect for the opposite reason – too much blood flowing to the lungs.

Treatment will depend on how much blood is getting to your child's lungs and being oxygenated. If there is insufficient blood flow to the lungs, then a number of shunts may need to be created, gradually allowing more blood to reach the lungs. These may include stretching the collateral and pulmonary arteries, or using stents to hold narrow arteries open. Your child's cardiologist will need to keep a close balance between maintaining his or her oxygen saturation levels, while protecting the delicate lung tissue from too high pressure from the left ventricle.

If your child's pulmonary arteries are very small, a series of shunts may be necessary, joining up the pulmonary arteries to a number of the extra collateral arteries. This procedure is called Unifocalisation.

These operations to increase flow of blue blood to the lungs are being improved all the time. If the right ventricle and the pulmonary arteries are of a good enough size after Unifocalisation, corrective surgery may be performed by closing the VSD and inserting a tube (conduit) with a valve inside it between the right ventricle and the pulmonary arteries.

This should get your child through two or three years of normal activity. After this time, you may find your son or daughter has started to slow down, may become breathless, and start avoiding stairs and other forms of exercise.

Further surgery can help by replacing the tube with a valve inside it by a larger tube because your child will have outgrown the original one.

It is not unusual for Arrhythmias to occur as your child gets older, and these can be treated with medicines or by Catheter Ablation. Long term follow up should allow these to be diagnosed and treated soon after they occur.

Pulmonary Hypertension of the Newborn

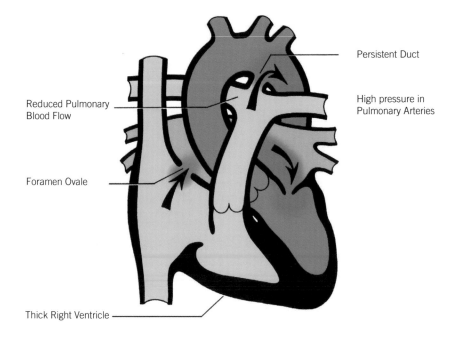

Persistent Duct

High pressure in
Pulmonary Arteries

Reduced Pulmonary
Blood Flow

Foramen Ovale

Thick Right Ventricle

At birth as the baby takes his or her first breath, the pulmonary artery has to start supplying blood to the arteries in the lungs for oxygenation. But sometimes the fetal circulation fails to convert to life outside the womb, so the arteries in both lungs remain as narrow and constricted as they were before birth. For this reason this condition is also called Persistent Fetal Circulation.

Because pressure in the baby's lung remains high (Pulmonary Hypertension), blue deoxygenated blood is directed across the valve (foramen ovale) between the right and left atriums and also across the duct (ductus arteriosus) between the two major arteries.

Although this is not a structural problem – the plumbing is all in order – your newborn will normally be referred to a cardiac unit for diagnosis. Treatment is by using medicines to get the lung arteries to open up, and if this is not successful, to use Extracorporeal Membrane Oxygenation (ECMO). This machine bypasses the heart and lungs, circulating oxygenated blood to your child's body while the fetal routes remain open.

Pulmonary Stenosis

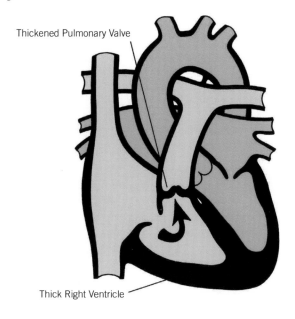

Thickened Pulmonary Valve

Thick Right Ventricle

Pulmonary Stenosis (PS) means that the valve which lets blood through to the lungs from the heart is narrow. The valve leaflets are thick and have restricted opening into the pulmonary artery. Because the right ventricle has extra work to pump blue deoxygenated blood through this narrow opening to the lungs, it may become thicker over time.

If your baby's valve is very tight, he or she may be noticeably blue, too breathless to feed and slow to grow and need treatment early on. Your child may be quite well when the PS was diagnosed – often the only symptom is a murmur made as the blood is forced through the narrow valve heard when he or she is examined by a doctor. The valve will be examined frequently to make sure that it is not causing problems – often a mild obstruction won't need treatment at all.

Treatments that are available are: stretching the valve without surgery - balloon stretching; stretching or replacing the valve using surgery.

Balloon stretching is low risk and often very effective. The procedure is performed under general anaesthesia (your child is asleep). The blood vessels at the groin are accessed in the same way as placing a drip or cannula and then catheters are threaded through veins to position a balloon into the narrow area. This is then inflated, to stretch the valve. The major advantages for this technique over heart surgery is that your child will have no scarring, and will be able to go home within a day or two of the procedure. Following this procedure, there is often a leak through the valve, but this is unlikely to cause any problems. The narrowing may recur in the future, in which case the balloon stretching can be used again, or your child may need surgery.

Sometimes surgery is the first option considered, or it may be offered after balloon stretching – this will be open heart surgery so the heart needs to be stopped and opened. The surgeon may be able to stretch the valve or free it to move more efficiently, or it may need to be replaced. The valve is removed and another valve (usually from a donor – called a homograft) is sewn into its place. Although these valves are very effective, your child will have to have regular follow up and a replacement may be needed within a few years.

Replacing a valve using a catheter is a procedure your child may be offered – the valve is inserted using a catheter to deliver it to the position between the right ventricle and pulmonary artery. At the present, this is more likely to be offered to older children and young people. Advantages over surgery are that the heart does not have to be stopped, the heart lung machine doesn't have to be used, so recovery is very fast, and you can expect your child home within a few days. The main disadvantage is if the valve doesn't work as it should, surgery will be needed. Long term follow up will be needed to check the valve function for deterioration, but whichever treatment your child receives, the outlook is good.

Reflex Anoxic Seizures

If your child has been diagnosed with Reflex Anoxic Seizures (RAS), you may know that any kind of sudden shock or pain (however slight) can cause your child to lose consciousness. This is because for some reason the vagus nerve is overstimulated and affects the sinus node in the heart and slows it dramatically causing unconsciousness. The unconscious period can last over an hour although it is typically for only a few minutes. Although these attacks can be very frightening, they don't seem to damage the heart or the brain in any way, and your child can grow out of them.

While there is a chance that an attack will occur, obviously you will need to forewarn anyone who is caring for your child in your absence, particularly in a situation where an attack is more likely. Cold water on the face is known to cause attacks, so swimming may be best avoided unless your child has one-to-one attention.

Unfortunately these attacks may have been misdiagnosed as epilepsy. Once RAS is suspected, your child will be taken off any medication for epilepsy and you may be asked to make a record of the attacks and when they occur.

If the attacks continue to affect your child badly or continue into teenage years, there may be a need for treatment in the form of a pacemaker to take over when the heart stops. Your child's GP can advise if this is an option and refer his or her case to a cardiologist at a specialist children's heart hospital.

Supra-Ventricular Tachycardia

Tachycardia means a fast heart rate. The most common kind in children is the kind that originates in the atriums and is called Supra-Ventricular Tachycardia, or SVT. Your child may have SVT diagnosed when being treated for another heart defect or after surgery. It is also possible for SVT to be diagnosed with no other heart defect being present, as a result of the baby or child appearing tired and breathless and uncomfortable.

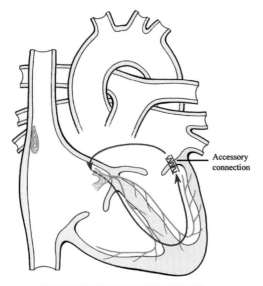

Accessory connection

ATRIO-VENTRICULAR RE-ENTRY CIRCUIT

Diagnosis might be by ECG over a period of time (Holter Monitor), a stress test or by an electrophysiology study, a diagnostic catheter test.

The SVT might be caused by an extra pathway, which allows the electrical impulse to travel in a circular movement causing the heart to race. If it can be seen on an ECG when your child is at rest, it is called Wolff- Parkinson- White Syndrome (WPW). An alternative name give to this is Accessory Pathway.

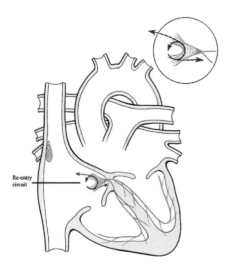

Re-entry circuit

ATRIO-VENTRICULAR NODAL RE-ENTRY CIRCUIT

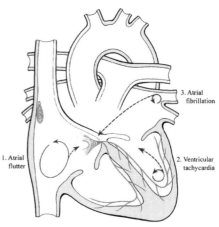

3. Atrial fibrillation

1. Atrial flutter

2. Ventricular tachycardia

OTHER RE-ENTRY CIRCUITS

WPW can arise spontaneously but it can sometimes be found in other family members, so you will be invited to have them checked out.

Another type of extra pathway may be in the sinus or atrioventricular node – although less likely in a child and difficult to see on an ECG.

Sometimes the Tachycardia is caused by a Re-Entry Circuit somewhere in the walls of the atriums, which start to produce rapid impulses. It can cause the atriums to contract chaotically and inefficiently, called Atrial Flutter or Atrial Fibrillation – this commonly occurs when the atriums are abnormal, either stretched as a result of being very large or as a result of previous surgery. Over time this can weaken the heart muscle.

How do you know your child is having an attack? If your child is young, you may be able to see a blood vessel in the neck twitching or fluttering. Your child may be pale and breathless and an older child may become irritable, and complain of an uncomfortable feeling in the chest or tummy. Most attacks of SVT are not likely to cause your child to be ill – he or she should recover as soon as it has finished, although this may be a matter of hours.

Once your child has been diagnosed, you will be given information on what to look out for and what to do. You may need a monitor to alert you if your child has uncontrolled serious attacks which last a long time and leave him or her weak and exhausted – your child's cardiologist should tell you if this is necessary.

With an older child, ask for written information about his or her condition to pass on to nursery or school.

Sometimes an attack can be stopped by putting a wet cold towel around the child's head. Older children can learn tricks to stop an attack by taking deep breaths, making their ears pop, putting a finger on the back of the tongue to make themselves gag, or drinking cold fizzy drinks quickly.

If there is a prolonged attack and the child seems in difficulties, you may be advised to take your child into hospital, so that medicines can be delivered straight into a vein (an intravenous injection). If this fails, an electric shock can be delivered to the chest while your child is under sedation or anaesthetic – this is called Cardioversion and should shock the heart back into normal rhythm.

Long term treatment is usually with medicines – these may need a while to adjust to the right dose and can have difficult side effects, but your child may not need medication for more than a year or two.

If these fail to solve the problem, a procedure called Ablation is often successful. After identifying exactly where the problem arises, a catheter is threaded into the heart to the area where the problem is caused, and the extra pathway are destroyed by heating up the muscle. This procedure is less likely to be used on a baby as the chance of damage to other tissues of the small heart are high. In an older child, there is still a possibility that the heart's own pacemaking ability will be damaged. In this event, your child would need to have a pacemaker implanted straightaway.

If there are no complications your child should only be in hospital for a day or two, and should be completely well afterwards.

Tricuspid Atresia

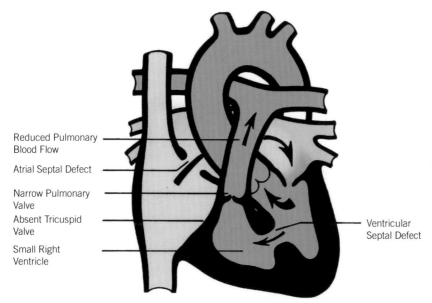

Reduced Pulmonary Blood Flow

Atrial Septal Defect

Narrow Pulmonary Valve

Absent Tricuspid Valve

Small Right Ventricle

Ventricular Septal Defect

Tricuspid refers to the valve on the right side of the heart which controls blood flow between the right atrium and right ventricle. Atresia means blocked or missing. With this condition, your child will have no way of blood flow to the lungs from the right atrium. Instead, blue deoxygenated blood returning from the body has to pass from the right atrium through a hole – an Atrial Septal Defect - into the left atrium. From here, it will be mixed with red oxygenated and pumped through the mitral valve into the left ventricle. The powerful left ventricle pumps blood to the body.

Your child may depend on a hole – Ventricular Septal Defect - between the left and right ventricle to allow some blood through to the right ventricle to reach the lungs, or the ductus arteriosus between the pulmonary artery and the aorta, which should have closed at birth, may still be open and carry extra blood from the left side of the heart to the lungs. Because blue blood mixes with the red being pumped round the body, your baby may look blue. The lack of blood flow to his or her lungs will mean that there is insufficient oxygen reaching the body for normal growth. Your child may be breathless and difficult to feed.

Treatment will involve increasing the amount of blood from left side of the heart into the lungs by creating a shunt. This can mean keeping the ductus arteriosus open with medicines, or making a larger hole in the wall between the atriums. Usually these can be carried out using catheter procedures. Sometimes a shunt is created using a plastic tube and surgically implanted between the aorta and pulmonary artery.

Once your child is bigger, operations to allow the blue deoxygenated blood to flow to the pulmonary artery - bypassing the right ventricle and pulmonary valve and sometimes even the right atrium – can be carried out.

These operations to increase flow of blue blood to the lungs – Fontan-style - are being improved all the time. The most common procedure is to attach the superior vena cava, the big blood vessel bringing blue deoxygenated blood from the upper body to the heart, directly to the pulmonary arteries to the left and right lungs. This operation is called the Bi-Directional Glenn Shunt.

This should get your child through two or three years of normal activity. After this time, you may find your son or daughter has started to slow down, may look bluer, become breathless, and start avoiding stairs and other forms of exercise. Further surgery can help when the blue deoxygenated blood from the lower body, carried by a blood vessel into the heart, called the inferior vena cava, is also connected to the pulmonary artery –this is called the Total Cavo-Pulmonary Connection.

During these operations to separate the circulation of red and blue blood in the heart, any existing holes between the two sides of your child's heart will be closed, perhaps leaving one small hole between the atriums – a Fenestration – to help the heart adjust to the change in pressures less abruptly. The hole may close of its own accord, or need closing using a catheter procedure later.

After these surgeries, because the blood is flowing more slowly to the lungs as it has no pumping impetus from the right ventricle, there is a danger of blood clots forming. Your child may be given either aspirin or warfarin – both act as anticoagulants to stop this potentially dangerous event happening.

The operations to improve (palliate) your child's condition do not correct his or her circulation, but should allow him or her to undertake most normal activities.

Occasionally many years later, Arrhythmias occur as your child gets older, and these can be treated with medicines or by Catheter Ablation. Long term follow up should allow these to be diagnosed and treated soon after they occur.

Transposition of the Great Arteries
Simple Transposition of the Great Arteries (TGA)

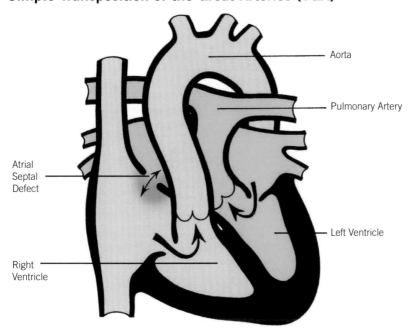

Aorta

Pulmonary Artery

Atrial Septal Defect

Left Ventricle

Right Ventricle

In Transposition of the Great Arteries (TGA), the aorta and pulmonary artery are plugged into the wrong sides of the heart – so the aorta takes blue blood from the right ventricle back round the body, and the pulmonary artery takes red oxygenated blood from the left ventricle back to the lungs.

If this heart problem wasn't spotted before birth, your child would have become progressively more ill, as the fetal circulation closed down in the first days of life. This closure results in the hole (ASD) between the left and right atrium becoming smaller. Its presence allows oxygenated blood to pass from the left to the right, through the tricuspid valve to the right ventricle and into the aorta, so at least some oxygenated blood reaches the body, so it may be necessary to increase the size of the ASD using a balloon catheter, before a repair is carried out.

The surgical procedure is called an Arterial Switch operation. In this, the aorta and pulmonary arteries are cut and reimplanted back into the correct sides of the heart. This is a far more complicated surgery than it sounds as the blood vessels are small. The arteries which take oxygen to the heart muscle (the coronary arteries) arise from the first part of the aorta and need to be reimplanted also, as without these the heart muscle cannot pump.

This surgery should result in a complete correction of the heart. There will need to be followed up to check the valves – they remain on the 'wrong' sides of the heart, and it is not unusual for the valve in the aortic position to develop a leak. Rarely the coronary arteries, become narrowed and may need further procedures to make sure they are efficient.

Complex Transposition of the Great Arteries

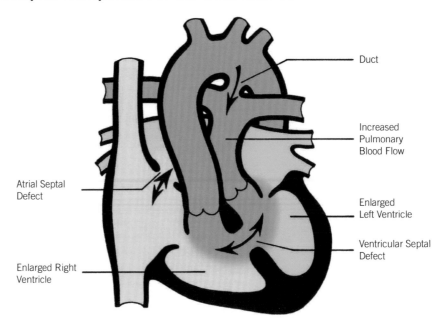

Duct

Increased Pulmonary Blood Flow

Atrial Septal Defect

Enlarged Left Ventricle

Ventricular Septal Defect

Enlarged Right Ventricle

In Complex Transposition of the Great Arteries (Complex TGA), the aorta and pulmonary artery are plugged into the wrong sides of the heart – so the aorta takes blue blood from the right ventricle back round the body, and the pulmonary artery takes red oxygenated blood from the left ventricle back to the lungs. Because there is a hole between the two Ventricles (VSD), blue and red blood mix and is pumped to the body and to the lungs.

If the heart defect wasn't diagnosed before birth, your child may have been blue, breathless and difficult to feed. The higher pressure from the left ventricle pumping to the lungs will have made your baby very breathless, unless he or she also has Pulmonary Stenosis – a narrowing of the pulmonary valve – which protects the lungs initially from the high pressure. Your child may be able to have the Arterial Switch surgery described under Simple TGA – the aorta and pulmonary arteries are switched around to the correct sides of the heart and the coronary arteries are reimplanted.

But with Complex TGA, the Arterial Switch may not be possible. Instead your child may have procedures to increase the mixing of blood, and to protect the lungs from increasing pressure. When he or she is older, sometimes the blockage between the heart and the pulmonary arteries can be bypassed using a tube with a valve in it (a conduit) inserted between the right ventricle and pulmonary artery. The VSD will then be closed so that the left ventricle no longer pumps blood through to the right ventricle. This operation is called a Rastelli Procedure. As the tube will not grow with your child, the surgery will be delayed until he or she is old enough to have a larger conduit inserted. Problems sometimes occur when the tube blocks, or when it becomes narrower and inadequate for the child's needs – they often need to be replaced after several years.

In some cases when the heart defect is more complicated, there may the option of a Fontan-style operation to take blue deoxygenated blood back to the lungs directly, bypassing the right side of the heart, using the left and right ventricles together as a single pump to send oxygenated blood to the body.

Truncus Arteriosus

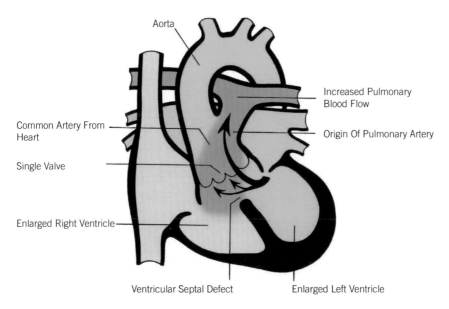

Aorta

Increased Pulmonary Blood Flow

Common Artery From Heart

Origin Of Pulmonary Artery

Single Valve

Enlarged Right Ventricle

Ventricular Septal Defect

Enlarged Left Ventricle

Truncus Arteriosus (TA) means that there is only one artery carrying blood away from the heart instead of two. Your child should have a pulmonary valve and pulmonary artery to carry blood to the lungs, and an aortic valve and aorta to carry blood to the body. Instead there is a single large valve, in place of the pulmonary and aortic valve, leading to one large single artery, which then divides into the pulmonary artery and aorta. There is also a large hole between the left and right ventricles: a Ventricular Septal Defect (VSD). You may be told that your child has type one, two or three TA, depending on where the pulmonary arteries arise. These defects result in a mixture of blue deoxygenated and red oxygenated blood being pumped to the body and there is a very high blue and red blood flow to the lungs, making your child breathless, liable to repeated infections, and poor weight gain. Medicines may help but open heart surgery is needed in the first weeks of your child's life to prevent high blood pressure in the lungs (Pulmonary Hypertension) damaging them permanently.

The flow of blue deoxygenated blood to the lungs will be separated from the red oxygenated blood to the body. Your child will have the hole between the ventricles patched, and the pulmonary arteries disconnected from the single artery. A tube with a valve in it (a conduit) will be implanted between the right ventricle and the pulmonary arteries. The large artery now becomes the aorta with the single valve as the aortic valve. This operation is called the Rastelli Procedure.

Problems that often occur after the initial recovery after surgery are leaking of the aortic valve, which may need further surgery or replacement to make it efficient, and Arrhythmias – the electrical system of the heart can be affected resulting in your child's heart beating too fast, slowly or irregularly. Arrhythmia may be treated with medicines, pacemaker, or Catheter Ablation. Long term the conduit does not grow with your child and will need replacing. Your child will need long term follow up to deal with any problems as they arise.

Ventricular Septal Defect

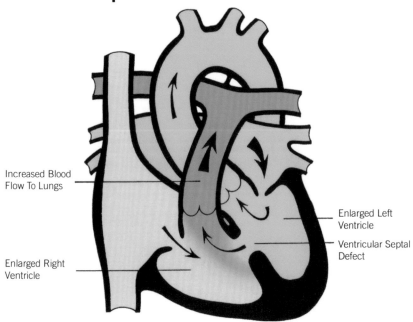

Increased Blood
Flow To Lungs

Enlarged Left
Ventricle

Ventricular Septal
Defect

Enlarged Right
Ventricle

A Ventricular Septal Defect (VSD) is a hole in the wall between the left and right ventricles – the pumping chambers of the heart. Because the left ventricle pumps blood around the body, it pumps at higher pressure than the right ventricle. This means that in most VSDs, some of the oxygenated red blood will be forced into the right ventricle, and from here will be pumped back to the lungs.

The amount of this blood flow depends on how big the hole is, and where it is. If your child has higher pressure than normal in the right side of the heart, blue deoxygenated blood may be forced into the left ventricle and, mixed with red oxygenated blood and, pass around the body.

A small VSD may cause no problems, and usually closes by itself over a period of time. Your child will be checked in outpatients to make sure that this is happening, and will be discharged by the cardiologist once the VSD cannot be detected. But if your child is unwell because of the VSD – too much blood flow to the lungs can make your child breathless with frequent chest infections, slow to grow and put on weight – treatment will be needed. This can be either medicine to help the heart until the VSD closes of its own accord, or closure of the VSD without surgery, or open heart surgery. If medicine alone is used, it will usually be of the kind to help the heart work more efficiently, and reduce pressure in the lungs. Lungs are fragile, and can be permanently damaged by high blood pressure (Pulmonary Hypertension).

In recent years cardiologists have been able to close some VSDs without needing heart surgery by using a catheter procedure. The procedure is performed using general anaesthesia. A small cut made in your child's groin and catheters used to thread guide wires into the heart and through the VSD. Using echo and dyes (Fluoroscopy) guidance, a device called an occluder is positioned and then expanded to close the defect.

Some children develop an abnormal heart beat (Arrhythmia) after the procedure which corrects itself in a matter of hours. A few children may develop Heart Block – the heart beats more slowly, as there is interference in the electrical pathways between the atriums and the ventricles. If it continues to affect the child, a pacemaker may be needed to regulate his or her heart rate.

There is often a leak through the VSD which reduces and stops of its own accord. Some leaking helps the heart to deal with the sudden change in pressures, so is not usually a bad thing.

The major advantages of the catheter technique over heart surgery is that your child will not need the heart-lung machine for the procedure, have no scar on the chest, does not need to be on a breathing machine (ventilated) afterwards, and will be able to go home within a day or two of the procedure.

Open heart surgery will be needed if the VSD is unsuitable for closing with a device: surgery on a tiny heart is obviously harder than on a bigger one, so your child may need to grow to a size where surgery is safer. Medicines to make the heart more efficient will help. If your child is too breathless to feed well, the cardiologist may refer him or her for feeding using an NGT (Nasogastric Tube) – a tube through the nose and into the stomach. This means that feeding is no effort, and extra calories can make growth much more likely. You can continue to feed expressed breast milk through the NGT, and to nurse your baby to help establish or maintain breastfeeding.

If your child is suffering from very high pressure in the lungs, he or she may need surgery to have a band placed around the pulmonary artery to reduce the amount of blood going to the lungs (Pulmonary Artery Banding). The heart does not need to be stopped for this operation, although a short stay in intensive care may be needed.

The band will be removed when the VSD is closed later. Surgery to close the VSD will be open heart surgery – a patch will be put over the defect.

There is a good chance of complete correction and discharge from follow up within a few months of the surgery.

Ventricular Tachycardia

Ventricular Tachycardia (VT) is a fast heart rhythm which starts in the right or left ventricle. This tends to have more serious consequences than a fast rhythm occurring in the atriums, as the heart cannot pump efficiently to the lungs and body. Your child may have been diagnosed as a result of dizziness and blackouts.

VT is a rhythm which can occur as a result of inherited conditions, such as Long QT and Brugada Syndrome, or complex heart disease, but it can also arise spontaneously for no known reason.

Once your child is diagnosed he or she may be treated with medicines or be fitted with an Implantable Cardioverter Defibrillator (ICD) which works as an internal defibrillator to shock the ventricles into normal rhythm should a VT occur. Long term follow up is of course necessary.

5. Treatments and Complications

This chapter describes treatments which may be offered to your child: feeding, medicines, catheter procedures and surgery.

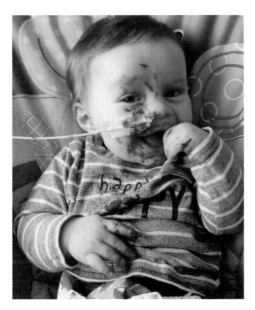

Feeding

It may be odd to think of feeding as a form of treatment, but for many parents it is the area where heart children need most input from health professionals. Getting enough calories into your child may be a necessary step to make him or her strong enough for surgery – so feeding is an important early step on the road to recovery.

Your child may have been diagnosed because of failure to gain weight – 'failure to thrive' - or you may have needed help feeding from the time your baby was born.

So why are so many heart children difficult to feed?

Some heart conditions cause children to be so breathless they cannot suck at the same time as breathing. Heart conditions can arise as part of syndromes which cause feeding difficulties where the structures of the mouth are not properly formed, where the oesophagus is narrow or compressed, or the stomach does not properly close. It is not uncommon for digestive problems to arise after surgery, or a period of nasogastric feeding in hospital to cause a child to lose the ability or will to feed orally. And a heart muscle labouring to get sufficient oxygen to your child's body needs more energy than a heart which doesn't have to work with defects in its system.

If you are struggling to feed your child and haven't been offered help yet, ask your health visitor or GP to put you in touch with a local pediatric dietician, or ask for help at your child's Pediatric Cardiac Unit.

Breast feeding: even if your baby cannot latch on, or suck for long enough to feed, expressed milk will provide the same nutrition, and will enable the supply to be kept going. If your baby is in hospital, you should be encouraged to breastfeed or express milk to be added to other feeds. If you cannot spend time at the hospital, expressing at home will be just as useful for keeping the supply going.

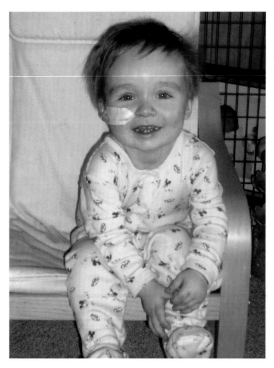

Solids: some children often have real problems being weaned onto solids, tending to gag on lumpy food and vomit anything that does disappear into the mouth.

Obviously it is important that he or she doesn't become dehydrated as a result of the vomiting so you may be advised to leave more solid foods for a few days before trying again.

Nasogastric Tube (NGT) feeding: for children who can't feed normally, or who need additional feeds, a tube can be threaded through the nose and into the stomach, where it can be kept in place for some time. Liquid feeds are then poured down so that there is no effort from the child. This can be very successful at getting the calories in there and adding on the weight. There are disadvantages: because he or she doesn't get hungry, the child may lose the need to feed orally, and it can become a long term fixture. The tube holds the entrance to the stomach slightly open, so there is a greater chance of reflux of feed – stomach contents coming back up. The tube can stimulate the gag reflex at the back of the throat, making it more likely your child will vomit. Some children enjoy pulling the tube out. Most parents don't enjoy putting the tube back in.

You will get help at home with supplies of feeds, and passing the tube. If you are using equipment at home for feeding, make sure that you understand where an NGT should be going and how you can tell – even if you are not passing it yourself you can keep an eye on it when others are.

Gastrostomy: this is a surgical procedure. An opening is made into the stomach so that food and medicine can be directly fed in. This is usually only considered after a long period of NGT feeding difficulty. Its advantages are that without an NGT your child does not look different, and he or she may find it pleasurable to start putting things in his or her mouth. The operation can be reversed. The disadvantages are that it requires surgery under a general anaesthetic, and can need time and care to heal.

If your child has severe reflux he or she will probably need a further operation to prevent the stomach contents escaping into the oesophagus (reflux).

Whatever your problem with feeding your child, another parent will have had it first. You may find that there is a mine of information on how to interest your child in food from a support group, and that you in turn will be able to help others with your own hard won knowledge.

Medicines

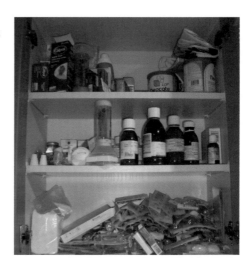

Many children will not require medicines for their heart condition at all, but in others medicines or drugs are used for a variety of purposes. These drugs are often prescribed to be given at home. The first time they are given will usually be by the hospital pharmacy, but after that they will be prescribed by your child's GP for you to get from a local pharmacy. Because some of the drugs are unusual for young children, you may find that this takes longer than normal (the pharmacy has to order them in) or the formulation is different (pills instead of liquid for example), or the entire name is different.

It is very important that you know how much of a drug your child needs, and how much of the made-up medicine holds that amount of the drug. If you are at all uncertain, query it with your pharmacist or with the Pediatric Pharmacist at your child's hospital. Some pills don't work as they should if they are crushed – so check before crushing them.

You may find that it is difficult to get syringes prescribed for your child – ask the Hospital Pharmacist or your Cardiac Liaison Nurse to write to your GP asking that, for the sake of accuracy and ease of administering liquid medicines, an appropriate size syringe should always be provided with liquid medicine.

An **unlicensed drug** is one which has not been licensed for use in children, but can be used in the absence of any that are as effective.

An **off-label drug** is one which is licensed for use in children but not for the treatment for which it has been prescribed.

A **side effect** is a reaction caused by the medicine unintentionally. These may be minor, such as slight rashes, or more important, such as nightmares and reaction to sunlight, or very serious, such as swelling of the throat.

Often there are twenty or thirty side effects for every medicine listed, and your child probably won't suffer from any of them. But keep a look out, especially when a new medicine is introduced.

The term **contraindication** means a situation when the medicine shouldn't be used – for example, if your child has been prescribed aspirin, it shouldn't be given if he or she is running a high temperature, and an allergy to eggs can exclude some forms of immunisation.

Your child may need one or more of the medicines described below, sometimes for a short time, for example before surgery, and sometimes for the foreseeable future.

Antiarrhythmic drugs: are used to regulate and strengthen fast or irregular heart beats – and include Verapamil, Disopyramide, Lignocaine, Mexilitene, Flecainide, Amiodarone, Adenosine and beta-blockers. If these are prescribed, your child may need to take these for the foreseeable future.

Antibiotics: Your child may need antibiotics for infections, which are nothing to do with the heart problem, or as preventative medicines, when they have health concerns such as no spleen, or a very poor immune system for other reasons. Around the time of surgery, antibiotics are used to avoid infections in the wound and especially to prevent infections interfering with the action of the heart and lungs. Bacteria which cause infections can become resistant to antibiotics over time, so it is important to limit their uses to those times that they are essential.

Anticoagulants: If your child has an artificial valve or had tubes implanted, or has a sluggish blood flow within the heart, there is a danger of blood clots forming and being pumped into the blood stream. To avoid this, anticoagulant drugs are prescribed. Warfarin makes the blood thinner by suppressing the production of Vitamin K in the liver. Because it is not a stable medicine, your child will need frequent blood tests (called INR test) initially to check that it is working properly, and regular less frequent tests later. The tests should ensure that your child does not bruise or bleed too easily. You may be able to get a home blood-testing machine to cut down on the number of warfarin clinic visits – ask your Named Nurse or Hematologist. Aspirin in small doses stops the platelets in the blood sticking together, and is a useful anticoagulant after a Fontan Procedure, in which the blood flows slowly through the right atrium. Currently new anticoagulants are being researched and may be offered to your child.

Beta-blockers: Propranolol is a commonly used beta-blocker, that reduces the rate and force of contraction in the heart muscle. It is useful in treating fast heart rates, high blood pressure and also reducing spasm of heart muscle in Fallot's Tetralogy.

Diuretics: When the heart is not working very well, water and salt accumulate in the body, liver and lungs, making the lungs heavy and difficult to expand. Frusemide and chlorothiazide are diuretics which make the kidneys pass more urine, getting rid of sodium, chloride, potassium and water. Spironolactone and Amiloride are weaker diuretics, which hold on to potassium. When these drugs are given, the lungs become easier to expand and less energy is used in breathing. Too much salt in your child's diet can reduce the efficiency of these drugs. You may want to give these medicines so that they work in the daytime rather than your child needing toileting in the middle of the night.

Digoxin: this increases the force of contraction of the heart muscle and slows down the electrical signal, so that the heart rate is slowed. It is used when the ventricles need extra pumping power, and also in the treatment of fast heart rates.

Immune suppressant: these drugs will be given to your child if he or she has a heart transplant, to prevent their own immune systems rejecting the new organ.

Vasodilators: drugs such as captopril and enalapril dilate blood vessels and as a result reduce blood pressure. They can be used in patients with high blood pressure to reduce it to normal. They can also be used in those patients with a normal blood pressure and a weak heart. Reducing the blood pressure reduces the work of the heart.

Invasive Procedures: Surgical and Catheter Procedures

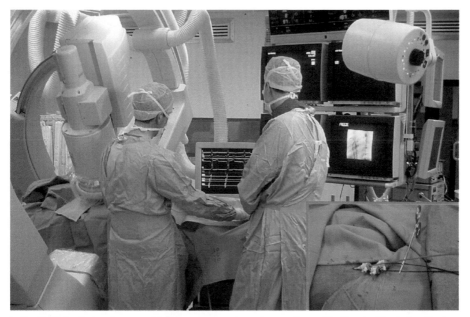

In the Catheter Laboratory, an ablation procedure is under way to modify the electrical circuitry in the patient's heart.

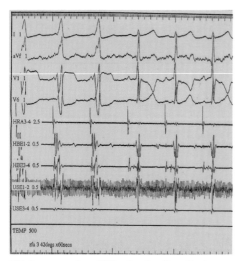

Ablation procedure ECGs showing the effect of the radio frequency pulses on the electrical pathways in the heart.

If this is a planned procedure (elective) you should have received information from the hospital well in advance of the planned date, explaining that there may be postponements, and telling you what to bring in with you, including your child's favourite toy or cuddly. There should also be clear information about where you can stay and how to secure the accommodation. Ring the contact number you should have if you are not clear on these points. No contact number? Call the ward or the cardiologist's secretary. You may also want to ask about help from the hospital play specialist with preparing your child for the procedure.

Your child may need to come in to hospital a day before surgery, although some pediatric cardiac units will offer a live-out option, so that preliminary tests are done on a day ward, and the child can go home or stay with you in hotel-style accommodation, until the night before the operation. The routine tests are performed to establish that your child doesn't have any infection which would be made worse by an operation, and scans will update the surgical team about the procedure to be performed. The anaesthetist may visit you to ask about loose teeth (don't want them falling out when the breathing tube is put into the mouth) and any symptoms of asthma or allergy.

The nursing team may ask the Play Specialist to help your child understand what is going to happen, and you will be able to see the intensive care unit if that is where your child will be taken.

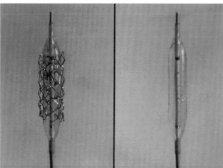

A balloon catheter (right) fitted with an expandable wire stent (left) will be inserted into a blood vessel to prevent it from narrowing again.

The parent's consent and the child's assent should be recorded (this may have been done at an earlier outpatients appointment) and you should be clear about what will be happening, and prepared for any risks attached to the operation.

Palliated or corrected: You may be told that your child's heart can be palliated or corrected. These terms are sometimes confused but generally **palliated** means that it has been improved but the

68

circulation is not fully corrected. Many complex conditions can be palliated but your child may never have a normal circulation. Hearts that are fully **corrected** have blue deoxygenated blood pumped to the lungs by a ventricle and red oxygenated blood to the body by another ventricle, without mixing. It does not necessarily mean the heart is 'normal' – there may be a prosthetic valve for example – but it functions like a normal heart.

Catheter Intervention: Sometimes your child's heart problem can be treated without medicines or surgery.

A catheter is a long thin tube which can be threaded through veins and into the heart, where it can be used to carry out small operations – such as stretching a narrow area using a balloon, closing a hole with a device, or destroying small areas of muscle.

Recently some valve replacements have been possible using a catheter technique rather than surgery. And some operations now use catheters and surgical procedures combined.

Catheter interventions are carried out in the Cath Lab within the children's surgical heart hospital, by a specialist electrophysiologist if the electrical system is being treated.

Older children may only need a local anaesthetic, whilst in others, sedation rather than a general anaesthetic is used. Because there is no surgical wound, the recovery time is a matter of hours, and once a check has been carried out to show the procedure was successful - devices are in place, leaking isn't a problem, or there is no Arrhythmia - you should be on your way home within a day or so.

Open Heart Surgery: Open (as opposed to closed) heart surgery means that the heart needs to be surgically opened, and to operate, the heart beat will need to be stopped. Obviously a period without the circulation of blood would be very damaging, so the work of the heart and lungs is taken over by a heart-lung bypass machine. Cooling to low temperatures reduces the need of the body for oxygen and protects particularly the brain from damage.

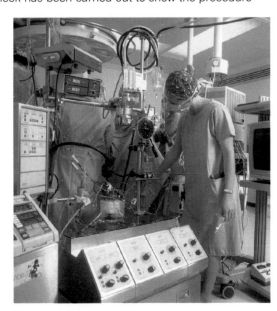

Heart-Lung By-pass machine.

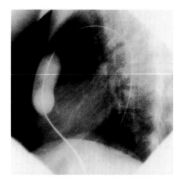

X-ray picture of a balloon catheter dilating a pulmonary valve.

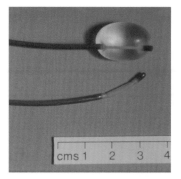

A balloon catheter for transposition.

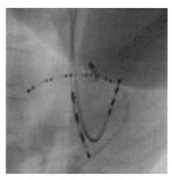

Left: X-ray of electro physiology wires being steered into the heart.

Blue blood coming back from the body is connected into the machine, which oxygenates it, removes harmful elements in it, and pumps it back into the child's aorta.

The period on the heart-lung bypass machine is kept to the minimum, and once the surgery on the heart is complete, it is given an electric shock to start beating again, and then the chest can be closed. Following open heart surgery, your child will be sedated and on a breathing machine (a ventilator) in order to allow your child to establish a normal breathing pattern. Because the lungs have been deflated during the bypass period, they also need to fully inflate to avoid infection, and the heart needs to establish a good rhythm after its enforced rest.

Your child will be in intensive care during this initial period of recovery – the length of time depends on the function of the heart and other organs and how slowly they adjust to the changes made by the surgery. It is often less than 24 hours but when complications or problems arise it could be several weeks.

Children who need a lot of care, but not one-to-one, may stay in a high dependency unit after moving from the intensive care unit.

Then it's back to the ward for a few days as your child recovers (probably faster than you will) and starts feeding normally, if a baby, or eating, drinking and running around, if an older child.

Closed Heart Surgery: If the heart doesn't need to be opened, the surgery is referred to as 'closed'. The heart does not need to be stopped, a heart and lung bypass machine isn't needed, and your child should be breathing by themselves in the recovery room after the operation. Most closed heart surgery won't need a period in intensive care, but this depends very much on the child's health and any complications that may arise.

ECMO machine: if a child is in severe cardiorespiratory failure, he or she may be attached to an Extra-Corporeal Membrane Oxygenation machine. This works like the heart-lung bypass machine used in open heart surgery, and takes over the work of the child's heart and lungs to allow them to rest and recover. Blue deoxygenated blood is drained into the machine, passed through an artificial membrane which acts like a lung to remove impurities and oxygenate the blood, which is then pumped into the aorta. This treatment can continue for several weeks, allowing the child the best chance of recovery.

Above: ECG recording from within the heart during ablation. Notice the changes to the ECG shapes in the top four traces. Radio frequency energy is shown by the bottom trace.

Catheter Procedures

Ablation: To ablate means to remove by erosion, melting, evaporation, or vaporization. A Catheter Ablation is a means of destroying an abnormal pathway in the heart which is causing Tachycardia - a very fast heart beat. This procedure is less likely to be used on a young child as the chance of damage to other tissues of the small heart are high. The exact location of the pathway has to be found first, using electrophysiological tests - fine electrical catheters are positioned in various part of the heart, the local electrical signals recorded and the fast heart beat is brought on. The exact position of the abnormal electrical connection can be pinpointed, and if it is a safe distance from normal pathways, an Ablation can be performed.

A catheter is threaded into the heart through a vein, and the small area critical to the heart rhythm abnormality is destroyed. This is via heat from radiofrequency energy. In areas at a greater risk of damaging surrounding tissue, such as the bodies own pacemaker, freezing (cryoblation) is used. There is a possibility that the heart's own pacemaking ability will be damaged. In this event, your child would need to have a pacemaker implanted.

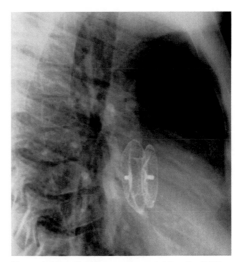

X-ray picture showing an expandable wire ASD device positioned in the heart.

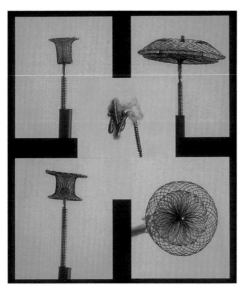

Balloon Angioplasty: Where there is a narrowing in a blood vessel, such as Pulmonary Artery Stenosis or Coarctation of the Aorta, balloon dilation may be used instead of surgery. A catheter is threaded through a vein and through the narrowed portion of the blood vessel. A balloon attached on the catheter is inflated and deflated in the area, so stretching it. This can be repeated at a later stage if the narrowing reoccurs.

Balloon Valvotomy: A valve that has narrowed (Aortic Valve Stenosis, Pulmonary Valve Stenosis) can mean that insufficient blood is being pumped to the lungs or the body.

Devices used to close holes and vessels using a catheter.

Even in very small babies, a catheter can be used to stretch the valve. A catheter is threaded through a vein or an artery, into the heart and through the narrowed valve. A balloon attached on the catheter is then inflated, deflated and removed, so stretching the valve and allowing more blood through it. If necessary, ballooning may be repeated several times until the child is old enough to have a valve replacement. It is usual for the valve to leak – called regurgitation – after ballooning.

This procedure has been used to open up an aortic valve in a baby before birth - when the valve is not working properly before birth, the left side of the heart does not develop and is more difficult to treat successfully. This is a very difficult operation with unknown outcome at this time.

Closure Atrial Septal Defect (ASD): Some ASDs – holes in the wall of the heart between the atriums - can be closed without needing open heart surgery by using a catheter procedure. The procedure needs general anaesthetic. A small cut is made in your child's groin and catheters and guidewires are threaded into the heart and through the ASD. Through the catheter a device called an occluder is positioned and then expanded to close the defect.

Closure Patent Ductus Arteriosus (PDA): PDA is part of the fetal circulation. If it does not close on its own, it allows some red oxygenated blood to be pumped back to the lungs, causing damage over time to the left ventricles and lungs. If catheter closure is chosen for your child, a small cut will be made in his or her groin and catheters used to thread guide wires into the heart and into the PDA. Using x-ray and dyes, (Fluoroscopy) a coil or plug is positioned and then expanded to close the duct.

Closure Ventricular Septal Defect (VSD): Some VSDs – holes in the wall of the heart between the ventricles - can be closed without needing heart surgery by using a catheter procedure. Most VSDs require surgical closure. Because there is high pressure between the ventricles, this is a more difficult operation than for an ASD closure. The procedure is performed using general anaesthetic. A small cut is made in your child's groin and catheters and guidewires are threaded into the heart and through the VSD. A device called an occluder is positioned and then expanded to close the defect. If this procedure causes an arrhythmia, as sometimes happens, your child may need to stay in hospital until it has stabilised for a day or two.

Stenting Blood Vessels: Narrow areas of blood vessels such as the pulmonary arteries, coronary arteries or the aorta, can be kept open by stenting. A stent is a mesh metal tube. When collapsed it can be placed on a balloon catheter, which is threaded through a vein or an artery and through the narrow area.

The balloon is inflated, so expanding the metal mesh, and as it is withdrawn and deflated the stent is left in place, holding the blood vessel open. Your child will need to be checked to make sure the stent has stayed in place, and follow up will be needed.

Pulmonary Valve Replacement: In adolescent and older children, it may be possible to replace a pulmonary valve using a catheter procedure. The valve is sewn inside a stent – a mesh metal tube – which is collapsed onto a deflated balloon on a catheter. The catheter is then threaded through a vein into the heart through the pulmonary valve to the pulmonary artery. Once in correct position the balloon is inflated and then deflated and catheter pulled back, leaving the stent with the new valve in place over the old valve.

It is not known how long these valves will last, as this is a fairly recent procedure, but it may save a large number of young people, who have undergone previous surgery such as the Ross Procedure, or for Fallot's Tetralogy, needing a further replacement surgery.

Fontan-Style Procedures

If your child has only one efficient ventricle, he or she will have mixing of red oxygenated and blue deoxygenated blood, and generally the same amount of pumping power to the body – which needs high pressure – as to the lungs – which need low pressure. Heart defects where these conditions exist are Pulmonary Atresia, Tricuspid Atresia, Complex Transposition of the Great Arteries and other complex conditions such as Hypoplastic Left Heart Syndrome. Little Hearts Matter supports children with these 'single ventricle' or 'univentricular' conditions - see page 148.

A Dr Fontan developed a procedure in the 1960s which separated red and blue blood, allowing all ventricular pumping power to be used to pump red oxygenated blood to the body and back to the heart, while blue deoxygenated blood flows directly back to the lungs. This has been improved over the years and may involve a number of operations to slowly change the increased pressures in blood vessels as they grow.

Original Fontan: Originally the right atrium was attached directly into the pulmonary artery.

Glenn Shunt: the superior vena cava, the big blood vessel bringing blue deoxygenated blood from the upper body to the heart, is attached directly to the right pulmonary artery so that the blood flows directly to the lungs. A Bi-Directional Glenn Shunt allows blood from the superior vena cava to flow into both the left and right pulmonary arteries.

Total Cavo-Pulmonary Connection: a tunnel is created through the right atrium so that blood from the inferior vena cava, the blood vessel bringing blue deoxygenated blood from the lower part of the body, is directed into the pulmonary artery.

Extra-Cardiac Fontan: a tube – conduit – is inserted on the outside of the heart from the inferior vena cava to the pulmonary artery.

Hemi-Fontan: Connection of the superior vena cava to both pulmonary arteries, similar to the Bi-Directional Glenn Shunt, and separating blue deoxygenated blood returning from the upper half of the body from that returning from the lower half of the body.

Fenestration: when pressure is raised on one side of the heart, a small hole is sometimes left or created to act as a pressure pop-off valve. It may close of its own accord or need to be closed using a catheter.

Konno Procedure

The Konno Procedure is an open heart surgery used when the passage to the aortic valve from the left ventricle is very narrow: Tunnel-Type Subaortic Stenosis. Thick muscle is cut away and the aortic valve removed – a procedure called Aortoventriculoplasty. Then the aortic valve is replaced using an artificial valve. The Ross Konno procedure is used if possible – then your child's pulmonary valve is transplanted into the aortic position and the pulmonary valve replaced - see Ross Procedure below.

Norwood Procedure

The Norwood is a complex surgical procedure, first used at the end of the 1970s, for babies whose left side of the heart hasn't developed – both the mitral and aortic valves are blocked, the aorta is very narrow and the left ventricle small.

During the Stage 1 of the Norwood Procedure when your baby is still very young, the big pulmonary artery is attached to the underdeveloped aorta. The aorta may have to be patched to make it big enough. This increases blood flow to the body. To maintain blood flow to the lungs a passage is made to carry blood from the newly created big artery to a branch of the pulmonary artery (a Blalock-Taussig type of shunt). An alternative to the shunt (Sano procedure) may be used to make a passage between the right ventricle and a branch of the pulmonary artery. The wall between the left and right atriums is removed so that oxygenated blood can move freely into the right atrium, and so through the original pulmonary valve into the newly created big artery (aorta).

Instead of the Norwood Stage 1, there is now an experimental procedure which is offered by a few centres, particularly in small or premature babies. It is called the Hybrid, because it uses both catheter procedure and surgery at the same time. A stent – a mesh tube which holds a blood vessel open – is inserted by catheter into the ductus arteriosus (part of the fetal circulation which connects the pulmonary artery to the aorta) and the surgeon puts bands around the pulmonary artery branches to increase blood flow into the aorta and decrease the pressure and the amount of blood going to the lungs. This is not as big an operation as it does not need open heart surgery or the heart lung bypass machine, but it is too early to compare its success rate with the more usual surgeries.

The second stage Norwood is either the Glenn Shunt or the Hemi-Fontan. As your child grows and becomes more active, he or she will need more energy, and at this stage, usually before the first birthday, a Glenn Shunt is performed. The big vein carrying blue deoxygenated blood back from the upper body to the right atrium is connected directly into the pulmonary artery. This means that more blue blood is reaching the lungs where it can be oxygenated and returned to the heart. Previous shunts implanted at the first stage of the procedure are removed.

The third stage Norwood aims to divide the circulation of the red and blue blood completely by directing the blue blood coming back from the lower half of the body in the inferior vena cava into the branch pulmonary artery, either directly, or through the divided right atrium, or externally to the heart through a plastic tube.

Rastelli Procedure

If your child has no pulmonary artery or a blockage between the right ventricle and a poorly developed pulmonary artery (Pulmonary Atresia) together with a VSD, the Rastelli Procedure may be offered. This involves fitting a conduit – a tube with a valve inside it – between the right ventricle and pulmonary artery. The hole between the ventricles (VSDs), which supplied the lungs with blood via the left ventricle, can now be closed. The surgery is delayed until a larger size of conduit can be used in an older child. It will almost certainly need to be replaced at a later date.

Ross Procedure

The child's own pulmonary valve (an autograft) is removed and transferred to replace a malfunctioning aortic valve. A donor pulmonary valve (a homograft) is then implanted in the pulmonary position. The advantages for this procedure is that the pulmonary valve is the same size and shape as the aortic valve, and being your child's own tissue should grow with him or her. The pulmonary valve will need replacing, but it is possible that this can be done using a catheter procedure.

Shunt

A shunt is an abnormal flow of blood, such as that which occurs if there is a hole between the two sides of the heart. Sometimes a shunt is created in the heart to improve blood flow to the lungs or body – such as increasing the size of a defect in the wall between the atriums in babies with Transposition of the Great Arteries.

Blalock-Taussig (BT) Shunt: used to increase blood flow to the lungs by attaching the artery to the arm to the pulmonary artery.

Glenn Shunt: attaching the superior vena cava – the blood vessel bringing back blue deoxygenated blood to the heart – directly to the pulmonary artery.

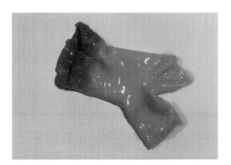 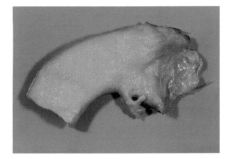

A homograft is a human donated valve. Left is a pulmonary homograft. An aortic/homograft is shown right. *Courtesy of Royal Brompton Hospital.*

Transplant

A heart transplant, replacing the child's damaged heart with one from a donor, is a form of treatment, not a cure, as the child, who receives the heart, will need to remain on medicines for the rest of his or her life. These drugs suppress the body's own reaction to the foreign organ, which is to try to reject it. Regular tests are needed to make sure that this process has not begun. See **Chapter 6 Heart transplant**

Unifocalisation

In some cases of Pulmonary Atresia combined with a hole between the ventricles (VSD), the blood vessels that should connect the heart to the lungs instead connect the lungs to the aorta. These blood vessels are called Major Aorto-Pulmonary Collaterals (MAPCAs)

Unifocalisation is a procedure in which the MAPCAs are rerouted into just one blood vessel (the pulmonary artery if there is one), which is then attached to the right ventricle using a tube made from human or artificial material. The hole between the ventricles is then closed.

Valve replacement

Valves that cannot be repaired may need to be replaced using insertion by catheter or open heart surgery. Homograft valves are usually used to replace the pulmonary valve. These have the advantage that they do not need the child to take anticoagulants to prevent blood clots forming, but they do need to be replaced after a few years - but see Pulmonary Valve Replacement above.

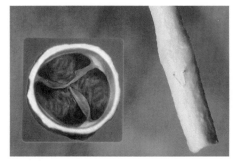 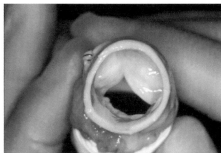

A conduit – an artificial tube and valve which is used where the patient's own valve is completely missing, or needs to be replaced.

A prosthetic (artificial) valve, is normally used in the aortic or mitral valve position. These can withstand the high pressure on the left side of the heart for many years, although it may need replacing if your child was small when it was first implanted and outgrows it, or if there are other problems, such as infection, inside the heart later. The main disadvantage of a prosthetic valve is that anticoagulants need to be taken to prevent blood clots forming. This rules out your child participating in contact sports, and he or she will need regular blood tests to check clotting times. You may find it easier to check your child's clotting times (an INR test) yourself, using a machine at home. Ask your Named Nurse or Hematologist.

In some cases a pulmonary valve can be replaced using a catheter procedure.

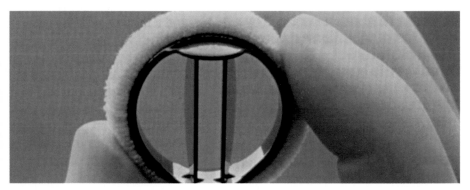

A Carbomedics artificial heart valve.

Devices

Implantable Cardioverter Defibrillator (ICD)

If your child has Ventricular Tachycardia, a dangerous heart arrhythmia, he or she may be treated using an ICD. This is a device which monitors the heart rhythm and administers an electric shock if it detects that the ventricles are not contracting (fibrillating). It also records the ECG so that the cardiologist can see the pattern of arrhythmia that emerges. The ICD, has a battery and electronic circuit, is implanted in the abdomen in smaller children, or near the shoulder and has a lead which is threaded through a vein to the heart. An electrode on the end of the lead is attached to the ventricles. The operation is not open heart, and can be done under sedation and local anaesthetic in older children. Recovery from this procedure is very fast, and your child should be out of hospital in a day or two. You must have written information about the ICD, what might affect it, and follow up appointments. The site of the implantation must be kept clean and dry and any sign of infection reported to the hospital.

Pacemaker

A pacemaker is a very small battery with an electric circuit, which is inserted under the skin, and one or two leads are attached to the heart. Although this may be done during the course of a bigger open heart surgery, it is usually carried out in the catheter laboratory. Replacement of the battery part of the pacemaker in older children can be carried out under a local anesthetic. Pacemakers can be put into newborns – obviously very important if your baby was diagnosed before birth – and the leads or battery parts need to be replaced as your child uses up the battery and as he or she grows.

Checks to find out how well the pacemaker is reacting and how much battery is left and changing the programme, so that the pacing speeds up or slows done, are carried out by sending electric signals from outside the chest. This is not a painful procedure, takes only a few minutes and can be done at an outpatient appointment.

The pacemaker battery lasts for some years – when it is running down, the box is replaced and is reattached to the leads into the heart. Leads may also need replacing at some future point.

Recovery from this procedure is very fast, and your child should be out of hospital in a day or two. You must have written information about the pacemaker, what might affect it, and follow up appointments. The site of the implantation must be kept clean and dry and any sign of infection reported to the hospital.

Ventricular Assist Devices

VADs are small pumps, which are inserted into one or both ventricles and attached to an external compressor, which provides the power. They help the ventricles pump blood and are often used as a bridging tool while a child is awaiting a transplant. You may hear them referred to as L-VAD. R-VAD, Bi-VAD (Left, Right or Bi-Ventricular Assist Device).

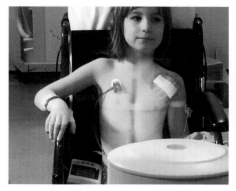 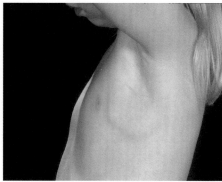

Site of a pacemaker.

Complications

Before your child has treatment, whether surgery, catheter or medicine, you must be told what outcome is expected (usually that your child will be better), and what side effects or complications are possible. As researching and testing of treatments improves, complications are less likely to occur, and those that do happen are treated quickly.

Catheter complications

Whether a test using a catheter, or a treatment delivered by catheter, this is an invasive procedure that, to be safe, relies on accurate threading of wires and tubes through the small veins and arteries of the heart of a child.

Arterial blockage: Arteries can develop spasm after a catheter is inserted causing a blood clot to develop. By blocking the artery, the clot could cut off the blood supply, so a drug such as heparin is used to disperse the clot. If this proves difficult it can be removed using a balloon catheter.

Embolus: small clots develop on the tip of the catheter, fly off into the circulation and can cause blockage of a small blood vessel. At worst this can result in a stroke – an area of the brain being deprived of blood. A drug such as aspirin helps stop blood platelets sticking together and heparin can be used to thin the blood.

Bruising: after the catheter is removed, the bleeding usually stops, but it may sometimes restart. As well as bleeding from the wound where the catheter was inserted, there can be painful swelling under the skin. The bleeding is stopped by applying pressure, but the leg can be stiff and the bruise takes a few weeks to disappear.

Device movement: devices, coils or plugs, are used to block abnormal blood vessels, or holes in the heart. Before your child leaves the hospital the position of the device will be checked. If it has moved out of position this may need to be corrected by catheter, or if this is not possible, by using surgery to remove the device and tie off the blood vessel or patch the hole.

Overstretching of blood vessels: a narrow artery can be stretched by a balloon catheter and it may then be held open with a a stent. If the blood vessel is stretched too far, the walls can leak, and surgery is needed to repair it.

Surgery complications

Blood loss: when the heart or its blood vessels are operated on, a large number of blood vessels are damaged. The surgeon will repair the larger vessels, and insert chest drains to allow any small amount of blood that collects in the chest to be drained away. After the operation, if a large amount of blood is drained, or if bleeding persists, more surgery may be needed to stitch up damaged vessels or the wall of the heart. Excess bleeding is more common in children who have had previous surgeries, as they will have grown extra blood vessels in scar tissue formed when recovering from the earlier operations.

Arrhythmias: sometimes during cardiac surgery the natural pacing mechanisms in the heart becomes swollen, resulting in an irregular or slow heart beat (Bradycardia). Temporary 'pacing' with the use of an external pacemaker may be necessary, and after most major heart surgeries temporary pacing wires will be put in place to allow for this. If the heart does not recover a permanent pacemaker can be implanted. Sometimes surgery can result in a very fast heart beat (tachycardia). While your child is in PICU, this may be treated by cooling him or her, and treating with medicines. If the fast heart beat continues, the child may stay on medication for some time.

Chylothorax: The thoracic duct is part of the lymph circulation system, which carries fluid including a high proportion of fat, around the body. If this duct is damaged during surgery, it can leak into the chest between the chest wall and the lung. This reduces the amount of space one or both lungs have to expand. The substance, which is a milky white, is chyle, and the condition is chylothorax. If this occurs, the child is put on a diet so that the fats are absorbed into the blood stream rather than into the lymphatic vessels. This typically takes up to four weeks but can be longer. Sometimes, the child will have to be on intravenous feeding so that the bowel is rested, which means a longer stay in hospital.

Paralysed Diaphragm: Sometimes during complex surgery in the chest, the phrenic nerve can be damaged or become swollen. This has an effect on the movement of the right or left diaphragm, which in turn affects the breathing pattern of the child. In children under one year, this can cause difficulties in weaning them from the ventilator. An operation to fix the diaphragm – to plicate it – may be needed to stop the abnormal movement.

Infection: Infection is always a danger after any operation. Because after open heart surgery the child is ventilated by an artificial airway, chest infections can be a problem.

These can be treated with antibiotics. Should the infection get into the bloodstream (septicaemia), a longer course of antibiotics might be required. An infection deep in the wound may need further surgery to clean it thoroughly. Some infections, such as MRSA, have become resistant to antibiotics and may need to be nursed in isolation. Although not a dangerous infection when carried in a healthy child, if it reaches a wound it can cause considerable damage.

Renal Failure: After a long operation carried out with the heart-lung bypass machine, the kidneys may not be able to excrete fluid and waste matter as well as they should. Following surgery the amount of urine your child passes is measured. If the amount passed is not sufficient, then Peritoneal Dialysis might be introduced. A fine tube is inserted into the abdomen and the peritoneal cavity is washed out with fluid. This draws out the impurities in the blood. A measured amount of fluid is inserted and then drained out each hour until the kidneys start working properly.

Vocal Cord Paralysis: The nerve supply to the vocal cord runs from the neck down into the chest around the duct between aorta and the lung artery before returning into the neck and the throat. It can become bruised and damaged by complex operations in the area of the large arteries. This can cause the voice to be weak and produce noisy and difficult breathing. In time, it usually improves.

Brain Damage: The child may suffer from fits and a period of loss of consciousness if the blood chemistry is abnormal – such as low blood sugar or calcium– or the brain does not receive an adequate blood supply - due to a blood clot, for example - or there have been convulsions due to a high temperature. The brain is very good at repairing itself and symptoms are often temporary, although sadly there may be lasting problems of more severe brain damage.

Tracheostomy: In a few cases children are unable to breathe without artificial ventilation - this can be due to an obstruction of the airways due to congenital defect or damage caused by heart surgery. A tracheostomy involves an incision being made into the windpipe to allow air to pass directly into it.

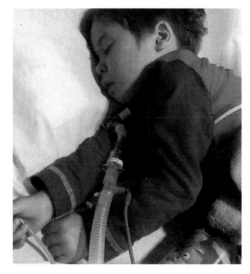

6. Heart transplant

Some conditions, such as dilated cardiomyopathy, can be life-threatening so quickly that transplantation has to be the treatment considered at a very early stage.

In other cases, such as single ventricle conditions, there may come a time when the cardiologist considers referring your child to another team in another hospital to see if there are other forms of treatment that could work. There may be a better drug that could be tried, or new operations that are proving successful. Hard as it is to put your child into the hands of another hospital team, this may be the best solution.

But if your child's health is deteriorating, life expectancy is limited and the heart looks like it can no longer be repaired or improved by medicines, you and your child may be asked if you want an assessment for a heart transplant. Where lungs have been damaged, assessment may be for a heart and lung transplant.

A new heart cannot cure your child – it is a treatment that demands a lot of medication, testing and dedication to outpatient visits. It is performed at only two hospitals in the UK, Great Ormond Street in London, and Freeman Hospital in Newcastle-on-Tyne, and you may have to be away from home for long periods of time. It relies on your child being otherwise healthy, and on a donor who is a good match becoming available. So it is not undertaken without a full assessment of the child's and the family's suitability.

The assessment

You will be asked to stay at the transplant hospital for around three days to be assessed by the transplant team – this can be made up of doctors, transplant coordinators, psychologist, social workers – anyone who will be involved with the decisions that need to be made.

There will be a number of tests (some of these may have already been carried out by your child's referring hospital)- usually heart and abdominal ultrasound, ECG to monitor the heart rhythm, check the lung function, sometimes a cardiac catheter to check pressures in the blood vessels. There will be blood tests – these are to check to see if your child is anaemic, whether there are viruses such as cause chicken pox present, and to look at kidney, liver and gland function. There are also important tests for donor matching such as blood group and tissue type.

Matching your child's heart

Blood group – if your child is more than 18 months of age, his or her blood group must be compatible with that of the donor. So which groups are compatible?
Your child's blood group is O, only an O donor will be a match.
If it is A, only O or A will be a match
If it is B, only O or B will be a match
And if your child is AB, then O, A, B and AB will all be a match

Tissue typing - some children will have been 'sensitised' – that is, have developed antibodies - to some other tissue type (because of blood transfusion for example), so this needs to be checked. The test, which looks at genes within the chromosomes, takes between 2-3 hours. If it is found that your child has been sensitised, it could be more difficult to find a safe donor. It may be possible to clean the blood of these antibodies to give transplant a higher chance of success

Size of the heart: The heart is a tight fit between the lungs, so the donor heart must be a good match in size. When heart failure occurs the heart enlarges - and it is very likely that a child awaiting transplant will be in heart failure. This can mean that a heart from an older child would be a fit.

A heart that is bigger than your child's own could squash the lungs and reduce the room for them to expand when breathing, and it could be difficult to close up the chest after the surgery. So a poor fit could mean a longer recovery. This must be weighed against the danger of waiting for a good fit.

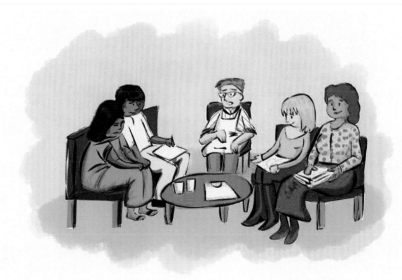

Informed consent discussion

Heart and lung matches - If your child needs heart and lungs, the size is even more important - lungs that do not have room to expand will not allow your child to breathe properly. The donor lungs can be reduced in size to be a better fit if there is unlikely to be another option.

The active transplant list

Once the assessment has been carried out, you will be told whether your child is being placed on the active transplant list.

The reasons for not being placed on the list could be
* that your child could not benefit from a transplant because he or she is not strong enough and the outcome would be poor. This does not mean that your child cannot be reassessed in the future if his or her general health improves.
* Your child is doing better than he or she would with a transplant, and can be reassessed
* Your and/ or your child are hesitant about undergoing the procedure, or are unable to consent

Urgent or non-urgent?

Non Urgent Category is for those who can wait at home with support from their usual hospital, and periodic appointments at the transplant centre – there may be 20-30 cases in the UK in this category. But if your child needs to be in hospital with intravenous treatment for heart failure or mechanical support, he or she will be listed in the Urgent Category – around four or five children will have this priority listing at any one time.

Mechanical support for a failing heart is improving all the time but the dangers are infection, bleeding and blood clots, which can cause strokes and long-term damage to other organs. **ECMO** takes over the work of the heart and lungs, often in an emergency situation. It is a treatment that will damage other organs with longer term use and is rarely used for longer than a month, but after a short period, when the heart has recovered a little, it may be possible to use other mechanical devices if a donor heart has not been found.

VADs (Ventricular Assisted Devices), such as the Berlin Heart, take over the pumping work of the heart. Sometimes even a very poorly heart (which is structurally normal) can recover full function after a period with a VAD, and of course the child could then come off the transplant list.

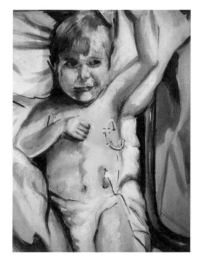

Awaiting transplant on milinerone

Waiting – It may be that your child improves with the support provided in the waiting period, and comes off the list, when a transplant would be less safe than keeping their own heart.

From the information above you will know that your child's chance of getting a transplant depends on many factors outside your control – state of health (urgent or non-urgent), size, blood and tissue-type status, availability of donated hearts, and priority. The guidance on who should receive donor hearts is decided by the NHS Blood and Transplant Board. When a heart becomes available, the heart is offered to the hospital with the most urgent case. If it is unsuitable, it is then offered to urgent cases, then to those on waiting list who may be suitable. In general, small children wait longer than older children. Sadly not all children will survive long enough for that special heart to become available.

Waiting at home

Apart from playing your part in keeping your child as well as possible, getting to hospital appointments, sticking to drug regimes, you also need to be in a permanent state of readiness. The transplant team will have told you how to contact them if you need to change your availability (because you are visiting relatives in another part of the country for example, or have changed your mobile number) and what you will need to take to the hospital. For the first few months, that may not be difficult, but then some of the detail may diminish- such as do you still have care in place for other children? They will not be able to accompany you. Is your phone always fully charged? Do you have your own medication readily available? Is the person who has promised to be your main contact with the outside world still in touch and has up-to-date numbers for concerned relatives and friends?

Your concerns over your child's state of health may be replaced by concerns over their state of mind. Children may decide to withdraw their consent – speak to the psychologist on the transplant team about how to deal with any fears and doubts, even if it may mean accepting your child's right to decide not to go ahead with transplant.

Most of us will realise that our wish for our child's recovery will be granted only when another family loses their child. It is not cruel to wish for the moment to come – you have no influence over the life of the donor – but it is human to acknowledge that others must suffer grief for your child to have a chance of life.

A child threatened with limited life expectancy, and still trying to live a regular life may develop behavioural problems. Siblings may find competing for your attention difficult and become overly demanding. Relationships may suffer the consequences of having this overwhelming priority in your life. Or you may find that the comfort and strength you draw from relatives and friends supports you and your family through this period, other demands are kept from you and you can approach the future optimistically. Take all the help you need when it is offered, and be kind to yourself.

There may come a day when you are at home with a post-transplant child who is fit and able, but used to receiving your concentrated attention and reluctant to take over their share of normal activities or relinquish their priority – may be worth finding out how to deal with this in advance.

The transplant team will know and understand that these problems exist for you, and may be able to help with contacts with other experienced transplant families.

The call to the transplant centre

Your centre will let you know how you should travel to the centre, and who can travel with your child – usually not more than two people can attend the hospital, but can travel separately.

There may be more than one call – you will be told to set off as soon as the donor organ is available, but before it has been fully examined. Your child may be ready and waiting at the hospital, but if the heart proves an unsuitable match, of course the surgery will not go ahead. You will have been warned of this, but it is a knock-back you may find hard to take.

Hopefully, the call will come, you will be ready to travel to the centre in the way you have been advised. And you will not be tempted to give your child anything to eat or drink even if the meal is on the table.

There is a limited time that a heart can survive outside the body, so bringing the child and the heart together in the shortest time possible, and under four hours essentially, is the aim of the recipient transplant coordinator, and the donor transplant coordinator As soon as you arrive at the transplant centre, you will be asked for your consent, your child will have blood tests and an xray, and given medicine to suppress his or her immune system (to prevent rejection of the new heart). Of course the heart is not removed until the donor heart has arrived and confirmed as suitable.

If your child is already a patient waiting at the transplant centre, and you are not staying at the hospital you will be called as soon as the surgery is likely, so that you can be asked for your consent, and of course to be as close to your child as possible during the operation.

After the transplant

First you should be kept informed when the surgery has been completed – this can vary, three to four hours but double that time if your child has had heart surgery before. This is because scar tissue will have formed which makes the heart more difficult to remove, and which is prone to bleeding. Your child's body will have been cooled before surgery, to help protect the organs, and once he or she is off heart bypass, a warming up to normal body temperature is started.

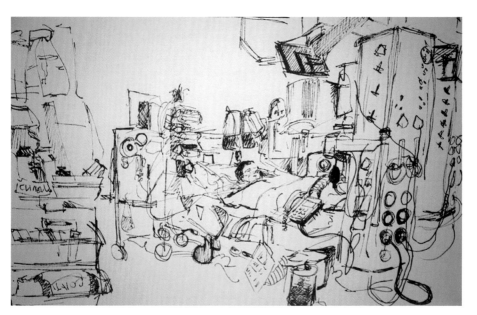

After transplant - equipment

Even when your child is transferred to intensive care, it may take some time to set up all the support and diagnostic mechanisms he or she will need. So it may be quite a substantial wait before you can be reunited.

The new heart can take a while to settle, and if it is not working effectively your child may be placed on ECMO, which will take over the functions of the heart and lungs, pumping blood and refreshing it with oxygen.

Either way your child will be heavily sedated, on a ventilator, tubes removing excess fluid from the chest cavity, and on drips to administer drugs and fluids. The heart may be swollen (or a little large for its new home) so the wound in the chest may not have been closed up. It will of course be covered to prevent infection. Monitors will keep a check on blood pressure and saturations, and all fluids going in and coming out will be measured.

You will have been told about the precautions you need to take to avoid your child getting infections, as their ability to fight them off has been much reduced, so this is a very dangerous time. For that reason, visiting will be limited to one or two people and may be stopped if there is a reason to think there is a danger of passing on an illness.

Recovery

How your child recovers depends on a great many factors, but a child who was very poorly before transplant will usually take much longer to recover than one who was in relatively good health. If yours is lucky enough to be the latter, you could be home within a month

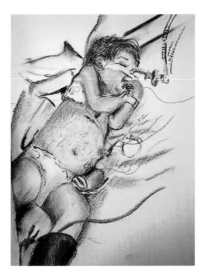

Sometimes a new heart will fail to function well after the initial period – in this instance your child will be given all the support available – ECMO, drugs and regimes to maintain his or her body in the best possible state. This is of course terribly hard on you and your family – weeks and months of waiting for the improvement that will last into the future. If your home life hadn't been severely disrupted before, it may be now. You may have to leave your child's bedside to sort out other aspects of your home life, and to support the emotional and practical needs of your children and extended family. All this is a heavy burden – again, accept any help that will free you from these responsibilities.

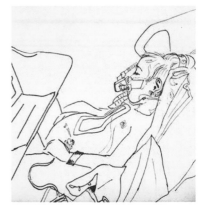

Without a good circulation over the period of the transplant, it is not unusual to have loss of muscle and as a result difficulty in sitting and walking. Some physiotherapy will be always be needed, and may continue for months or even years. Kidneys may suffer some damage, and dialysis may be needed for a time. Children who had difficulty eating prior to transplant sometimes need ongoing nasogastric feeding, through the nose into the stomach, or sometimes a gastrostomy so that they can be fed directly into the stomach.

Medicines

A CVC (central venous catheter)is usually put in place at the time of the transplant so that it is easier to take blood for testing and to deliver drugs directly into a vein. A Hickman Line or Portocath can also be used – this may be discussed with you and your child before the operation, to decide on the most acceptable site

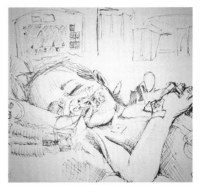

Long recovery

88

and they may still be in place when your child goes home. You will be taught how to use the device, and how to keep the site and spot signs of infection.

The medicines used will vary according to what becomes available, how your child responds. Use of these and how they should be taken will be discussed with you and your child at length. Achieving the best results means finely tuning dosage, and it will be one of your ongoing tasks to ensure the drug regime is maintained, even when your child feels completely well and tires of being 'medicalised'!

These are just some of the types of medicines used:

Antibiotics – are given at the time of the transplant. Young children may not develop immunity to common infections and may need to take antibiotics to anticipate and destroy infectious agents – prophylactics – for several years. Otherwise they are taken for the first three months, and afterwards only when a non-transplanted child would need them.

Immunosuppressants – these are drugs used to damp down the child's system's attempts to reject the heart. They are used singly or in combination according to how often rejection occurs and are balanced to prevent rejection while causing minimal side-effects. Steroids are used in older children or where rejection is hard to control
Diuretics – these are used to help the kidneys pass urine
Antihypertensives – to control blood pressure
Statins – to prevent high cholesterol and inflammation of the blood vessels

Home

You are home! Your own bed, and your own bathroom, but life will not be normal – the medication regime will be hard to get to grips with, let alone using feeding methods and diets that are not familiar to you nor to your child, and keeping sites free from infection - all can add foreign elements to routines (and use up large swathes of your time). And life will be punctuated by frequent visits to the transplant centre initially, and then to a local hospital which may be involved in shared care with the transplant centre and take over the more routine tests. So during the first three months, when the chance of rejection of the new heart is at its highest, and infection as a result of reducing your child's immunity most likely, visits and tests may be weekly. After a year, it may be every six weeks. During these visits your child will be examined for signs of rejection, irregular heart rhythms, and high blood pressure. They will be checked for infection and any side effects of the medicines they are taking, including early stages of cancers that can arise when immunity is suppressed.

Unfamiliar

Because transplant is rare in children, you are unlikely to have friends or neighbours living nearby who understand what is happening. You may very well have a community of families you have met at the transplant centre or through social media groups used by transplant families which you depend on for your social life. For practical support- the transplant centre or your local hospital should have provided details when you were discharged initially of where you could get help with respite, if necessary; services of community nurses to help with medical supplies; and to help you secure any benefits you are entitled to.

And lastly, transplant has been a successful treatment for many children, but the road getting there can be arduous, and once achieved it is not the Holy Grail – it can be the start of another difficult journey to reestablish family life while seeing your child through another set of traumatic health issues.

See **Chapter 13 Sources of help and support** for details of organisations that may be able to help out.

The copyright and intellectual property rights for the illustrations in Chapter 6: Transplantation are vested in Willow Langdale-Smith and are reproduced here with her kind permission

7. Communicating, consenting, concerns and complaints

In earlier chapters you may have learnt about your child's heart problem, and what treatments are available. Now we are going to look at how you as a parent are involved in ensuring your child's best interests during treatment.

You will want your child to get the best possible treatment for his or her heart condition, and to know that you have done everything possible to achieve that. But if you have looked through the earlier chapters you will know that pediatric cardiology is a complex area, with complicated vocabulary to get to grips with.

However controlled and composed we may appear to be, knowledge that our child has a heart problem and may need life threatening treatment creates emotional turmoil. And here we are having to learn a whole lot more about human biology, on a learning curve like a roller coaster, while dealing with a sick child, distraught partner, anxious relatives and often a nervous employer.

First you will have to get to grips with the more mundane problems. Assuming your child wasn't first referred to a heart hospital at birth, or as an emergency, the referral would have been made by your GP. In that case you may have to take your child either to a clinic run by a local hospital, or to a hospital specialising in children's heart problems.

Before you attend, check on transport and car parking. There is often a considerable distance between parking and clinic, so best to be dropped off, and let someone else park the car. Sometimes clinics give appointment times, and then add that you need to arrive an hour earlier for tests or registration – make sure you know when you have to be there! The clinic staff will make an effort to be prompt and efficient, but there may be waiting time caused by patients or clinicians. Be prepared – take food and easily managed toys.

Whenever you attend an appointment, it is useful to take a list of written questions and another person (and obviously the child). There should always be an opportunity, perhaps after the child has had an echo or some other diagnostic tests, to talk to the named nurse or the consultant cardiologist about the outcome. And make a note of the cardiologist's name – this is the person who is in charge of your child's treatment for the heart condition.

Whereas most people have a long view of their child's prognosis (will he or she be able to play football, drive, have children?) you may find that the consultant's view is of the immediate future – how the heart condition can be treated, what will be said to the GP and when another appointment will be needed for further assessment or treatment. A Named Nurse, who specialises in helping families and children, should be available, or will be on the end of a telephone if you want to discuss things in detail. Writing down your questions can ensure that you remember to ask them while dressing/ undressing and pacifying your child, gathering up bottles, snacks, outer garments, buggies and toys as you move around the clinic.

Taking another person can mean that you have a second pair of ears to hear what is said, even to make a note of it. There is often an opportunity for a discussion with the consultant alone, if the child can be occupied with grandma for a while.

Particular areas you may want to be clear on is whose responsibility is it to make appointments with, for example, a dietician if your child needs to put on weight before surgery, or the psychological service to help your child come to terms with their condition? If your child has problems which may not be related to the heart condition, make sure you know who you should be approaching – this is most probably your GP who will refer you to the pediatrician in your local hospital.

You should be given some kind of permanent record of the clinic visit, including a copy of the letter to your GP. If you cannot understand this (not many of us can), best to ask your named nurse, who should have been at the clinic.

Consenting

Before a doctor, nurse or therapist can examine or treat your child, they need consent or agreement. Before your child's medical records can be shown to an auditor, the patient or carer's consent is needed, and before your child is involved in a research study, the parent or child should consent, and the child's agreement (assent) must be sought.

This looks like quite a lot of consenting…

A couple of words of warning here – if you are the child's father you can exercise parental responsibility – that is sign the consent form – if:

- you were married to the child's mother at the time of the child's conception, or birth, or
- you are married to the mother now , or
- you are not married to the mother but your child's birth was registered on or later than 1 December 2003 and you are on the birth certificate

So generally only the child's mother and her husband can consent, unless the child is in care when the local authority has parental responsibility. Parental responsibility can be given to other people: a solicitor can provide a form which the mother and the other person will need to sign in front of an Officer of the Court or Magistrate, or a birth certificate can be reregistered with the father's name on it.

Consenting to testing and treatment

We tend to think of consent as signing a form to say that our child can undergo surgery – often a very hard and emotional task – but in fact any form of examination or treatment needs parental consent. Of course you are not asked to sign a form every time a stethoscope is applied to your child's chest, but in that example you are consenting by taking your child to the doctor, or encouraging the child to lift a vest. It is reasonable to expect the doctor to give a reason for the examination both to you, and your child if he or she is able to understand.

This principle extends to all other forms of test and treatment. You should have some understanding of what is being done and why it is being done, and so should your child, before you can be said to be giving informed consent to any test or treatment your child has.

Consent to treatment which may have some risks attached to it – for example a catheter or surgical procedure – is a process. You should have had time to take on board what the treatment will involve, what the outcome is hoped to be, what the risks are, and what alternatives there may be. In some cases there must be written information given to you – about a procedure that is new for example. You should have had time to frame questions that need answering. Your child should have received an explanation which is appropriate to his or her age and understanding.

You can see a website showing how many similar procedures to your child's the hospitals have carried out, and how successful they were. Before consenting to treatment you may want to seek a second opinion about the diagnosis, and the kind of procedure which is thought best, from one of these hospitals.

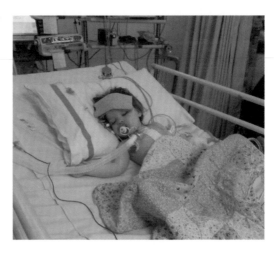

This consent process cannot happen in its entirety when there is an emergency, but even so you must have an opportunity to make a decision based on information and in your child's best interests.

At the end of the process, you will be asked to sign the consent form.

It's a good idea to involve children as much as possible in the consent process. Even when they're not old enough to make decisions completely on their own, children should still play a part in decisions about their health care.

Once children reach the age of 16, they can agree to examination or treatment just like adults. People providing health care do not then have to ask you for consent as well. A young person over 16 cannot be treated against their wishes.

A mother under the age of 16 has responsibility for consenting on behalf of her child, but her parents consent if she is the patient. But even children under 16 may be able to give consent for themselves, provided they are mature enough to understand fully what is involved. There is no hard and fast rule as to whether you or your child gives consent. A lot depends on the seriousness or difficulty of the proposed treatment. Although your child might be grown-up enough to consent to a vaccination, for instance, it might be too much to expect him or her to grasp all they need to know for consenting to a heart operation.

If you do not consent to treatment which health care professionals believe is crucial for your child, a court may be asked to help to decide. You may be able to go to court to request or prevent treatment, if you think it's in your child's best interests. Obviously going to court should be a last resort for both sides as it is enormously stressful for all those involved, especially if there is an older child who has some idea of the implications of the outcome. Make sure, as a parent, you have a thorough understanding of what is being proposed, and that you have given your child's clinical team an opportunity to talk through what troubles you about it.

Even if your child is grown-up enough to give consent independently, people providing treatment will still encourage them to involve you in their decision. But if a child refuses to share information with parents, normally health care professionals must respect their wishes.

Consenting to identifying your child for audit

When they visit the hospitals to collect and check information, the auditors need to review some medical records chosen at random. So when your child next goes into hospital for a procedure you (or your child if he or she is old enough) will be asked to give written consent for the medical record to be seen. This is not the same as consenting to treatment.

Consenting to research

There is a good chance that as the parent of a child with a heart condition you will be asked to consent to your child being recruited into a research study at some time. Areas of study connected with genetics, the best forms of medicine, intensive care equipment, and surgical procedures are all desperately important to improve the future for children – although it may never be an advantage to your own child. The research could be to compare two different kinds of medicines or surgical procedures for example, or it may be just looking at blood samples with no relevance to your child's treatment.

If your child is asked to take part in a research study, you must be given an information sheet (and your child a sheet appropriate to his or her level of understanding). Before your child is asked to participate, the research will be approved by a Research Ethics Committee, which will particularly look to see that there will be no harm to your child, and that confidentiality will be observed. You should both ask as many questions as you want before coming to a decision, for instance about the purpose of the research, the risks and benefits there might be, and what feedback you will get.

It is as well to know that a drug which benefits your child during a research trial won't necessarily be available to him or her once that part of the study is completed. In 'blind' trials you will not be allowed to know which type of drug or procedure is being used on your child, as the basis of the research is to make sure there is no prejudice in assessing the results.

With your consent, your child will be asked to assent from an early age and is, as you are, entitled to pull out at any stage in the research project.

If you or your child decide not to take part or continue in a research study, this must not be allowed to jeopardise the ongoing care he or she receives.

Deferred, or without prior, consent: In some cases treatment which is part of a research study may have been given to your child before consent has been requested – emergency treatment for example. You should be given all the information at the earliest time and be in a position to give your consent or to withdraw your child and any of his or her medical records entered into the research.

Second opinion

When deciding about consent– and assuming that life-saving emergency treatment is not being delayed – you may want to consider asking for a second opinion from another cardiologist or surgeon from another hospital about your child's diagnosis or treatment.

First it is important to know that hospitals which are allowed to carry out treatment for children's heart conditions are very closely monitored. For information on the success of the procedures similar to that which is being proposed for your child check with Children's Heart Federation, or British Heart Foundation to find the information for you. This will give you an idea of the number of similar procedures the team at the hospital have carried out successfully. **See Chapter 13 Sources of help and support.**

Second, remember that decisions about treatments are made jointly by several senior clinicians, not just by one person alone.

You have a right to **ask** for a second NHS opinion, but no legal right to get one! So it is as well to look very carefully at the information you have been given, and talk to the cardiologist or surgeon or your named nurse as to why you are thinking about it. You may have had poor information, or heard from another parent that a treatment not offered to your child is available at another hospital.

Before pursuing a second opinion it would be useful to know if the clinicians have already taken one from elsewhere, as they sometimes do when they know of a colleague who has had similar cases. Some surgeons and cardiologists build up expertise in procedures, particularly new ones. Ask if you think this could apply to your child.

Taking a second opinion could delay your child's hospital treatment, although you should be able to rely on the clinicians that no harm results from your request. Expect to discuss any concerns you have with the staff – there may have been a misunderstanding. Always remember that they are the experts and as human beings they will respond best to your polite enquiries rather than confrontation and accusation. So you will be saying 'I am thinking about getting a second opinion as to which is the best form of treatment for my daughter' rather than 'I want a second opinion because I don't think this hospital is good enough' for example.

If, after carefully talking any issues through with the staff, you want to have a second opinion, either your child's cardiologist or your GP can agree to make the referral. Your child's records and test results will be sent off, and once a second opinion is given, you may want to move to the new medical team or stay where you are.

Concerns and complaints

For most families, diagnosis, treatment and recovery of their child are straightforward. Of course there is anxiety and the odd hiccup along the way, but these are quickly resolved by the normal means we have at our disposal. So what happens when it looks as if things are going wrong? In this strange new world that you inhabit, it may be more of a problem to know how to tackle concerns that you have.

However annoyed, upset or frightened you are, try your hardest to avoid confronting staff with accusations. 'Don't you dare come near my child without washing your hands' may be better phrased as 'I think you've forgotten to gel/wash/glove your hands'. When a serious problem may have arisen, it will be almost impossible for people on the spot to explain what has happened, or to apologise if appropriate, immediately. Ask for an explanation within a day or two, in writing if you want to assess it carefully.

Keep your local patient liaison service informed at all stages: this is PALS in England, the Community Health Council in Wales, Local Health Council in Scotland and Social Services Council in Northern Ireland. Below we are quoting frequent problems that people have to deal with and how to deal with them:

I can't understand it

How stupid do you feel when being given very important information, you've already said 'what does that mean?' three times in the last two minutes? Once an explanation has come to an end, one technique is to say 'So can I just check ... you are saying that ...?' Another way is to ask how to spell particularly strange words and then check what they means.

The patient has PA with VSD and mapcas, tricuspid regurgitation velocity of 3.5/sec and LV EF of 22%. ECG substantially normal ... nonconfluent pulmonary arteries.. potential for unifocalisation ...

You are allowing the person giving you the information to explain as clearly as he or she should have done in the first place.

Some hospitals are making a great effort to translate their letters to GPs into straightforward language, but if you can't understand it when you see the copy, contact your Named Nurse and ask what it means.

They didn't tell me

Some kindly clinicians think it is all too much for us to deal with, and may keep back information. Problem is that when we find out we haven't been told, it is difficult to trust staff again. (And there again, there are some parents who do not want information, and turn a deaf ear to what is said.) If you discover that you haven't been given information about your child's heart condition or treatment for it – for example, the GP letter hasn't been copied to you – first make it clear that you weren't told at the appropriate time, and then record in writing to your child's cardiologist that you want all such information made available to you.

If you yourself would like to see your child's medical records you may need to put the request in writing to the medical records officer or patients' services manager. You can see part of the records, or get a copy of the whole – that may take up to forty days and cost up to £50 for manual records ie not computerised.

I haven't been sent an appointment

If you expected to get an appointment and it hasn't turned up in good time, contact the clinic or the consultant's secretary and ask if your child's appointment has been overlooked or gone missing. At the end of each outpatient appointment or period as an inpatient ask if you need to make an appointment before you leave. Carry all appointments with you in a convenient small size diary which includes a next year planner, so that you can enter appointments for six months' or a year's time.

Encourage older children to make a note of appointments so that they avoid clashes with other aspects of their lives, if at all possible.

Our appointment has been postponed at the last minute - again

If a postponed appointment ruins a holiday, jeopardises employment and disrupts a whole family raise it with your GP, especially if this is the second occasion. Express concern and point out what problems have been caused by the change of appointment to the clinic, or consultant's secretary. Put it in writing and copy to the hospital's patient liaison service. But if deterioration in your child's health is in question, talk to your patient liaison service and raise the possibility with your GP of transferring your child to a hospital where prompt treatment may be received.

Rudeness

Incidents of rudeness in hospital should always be reported using the ward manager and patient liaison service in the first instance and the complaints procedure of the trust subsequently. If you feel that you or your child were vulnerable to careless words rather than rudeness, point it out. Staff may not always be aware how easily feelings are hurt in these situations. If you want to complain about a service you receive at home, from your health visitor or community nurse for example, contact your Clinical Commissioning Group. Keep a record of anything that is said so that you can refer to it accurately later if need be.

Complaint about treatment

Complications can and do arise as a result of treatments with drugs and oxygen or invasive procedures – like catheterisations and surgery – and most of us will be aware that open heart surgery has risks attached to it. Largely the risks will be related to how complex your child's condition is, how long he or she remains on bypass and later in intensive care, how long ventilated.

Before you give consent you should be informed about the most likely risks of these treatments. But you may find that an unexpected hazard occurs which you believe may have been avoidable. Try to talk to the ward manager or charge nurse about what happened. You can also talk to the patient liaison service. Most of us want to know why it happened, and that steps have been taken to prevent it happening again. The patient liaison service will be able to explain how to take a complaint further if you wish to.

8. When your child is a hospital patient

Sometimes babies are taken straight to a Special Care Baby Unit after birth while awaiting diagnosis, or to a children's specialist heart hospital if the heart condition was found before birth. Or your child may need an admission when he or she is older for an invasive procedure – catheter or surgery.

The Children's Specialist Heart Hospitals

Children's heart conditions are treated in hospitals which have specialist children's heart units. Within the UK there are currently five such hospitals which don't offer children's heart surgery – they are in: Belfast, Cardiff, Edinburgh, Manchester and Oxford. Hospitals where children's heart surgery can be carried out are in Birmingham, Bristol, Glasgow, Leeds, Leicester, Liverpool, London, Newcastle and Southampton. Children in Northern Ireland are usually treated in Dublin.

So depending on where you live, you may have to travel a considerable distance to take your child for outpatient appointments, tests or surgery. Once your child has been referred to a specialist hospital, his or her cardiologist may hold a clinic at a hospital near you that you can attend as an outpatient. Even if there is a clinic locally, you may still have to go to a specialist hospital for some tests. Usually the specialist hospital may be the nearest to you but if it doesn't carry out surgical procedures you may be referred directly to another which does, for the period of surgery. All hospital staff you come in contact with will have an identity badge with their name. You may meet:

Anesthetist: is a doctor who administers drugs so your child is free of pain during and immediately following operations and catheter procedures. An anesthetist may also look after the ventilation if at any stage your child needs help with breathing.

Cardiac Liaison Nurse or Cardiac Nurse Practitioner or Cardiac Outreach Nurse: your Named Nurse, a senior nurse who specialises in helping and supporting heart children on the ward and when they are at home. You should be given the number to contact your Named Nurse if you have concerns when you are at home.

Catheter Lab Technician: is the person who records the pressures and maintains the equipment for the cardiac catheterisation procedures.

Chaplain: there are representatives of the main religious denominations visiting. To see one of them, just ask your ward sister or charge nurse.

Dietician: is the person who will advise on what and how to feed your child, should there be any problem with the normal diet.

ECG Technician: is the person who makes an electrocardiographic recording of your child's heartbeat and will be involved in the follow-up and checking of pacemakers.

Intensivist: is the lead doctor who will look after your child when he or she is in intensive care.

Matron: this is the most senior nurse, who makes sure your child has good nursing standards.

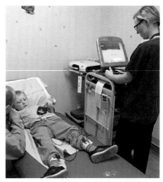

ECG technician

Pediatric Cardiologist: is your child's consultant and the person in charge of his or her or her care in the PCU as an in or outpatient. Some cardiologists specialize in particular aspects of diagnosis or treatment. Electrophysiologists are cardiologists with skills in the electrical workings of the heart, and can carry out catheterisations. Fetal cardiologists deal with the diagnosis of heart defects before birth. Cardiologists use the title Dr.

Pediatric Cardiac Surgeon: is a doctor especially skilled in children's heart surgery. Although you may not have met the surgeon prior to your child's admission, he or she will be familiar with your child's heart through discussing tests with the cardiologist and deciding when to operate. Usually he or she will meet you prior to the operation to explain what needs to be done, before you are asked to sign the consent form for the surgery, and once your child is out of theatre to say what has been done. Surgeons use the title Mr, Mrs, or Miss.

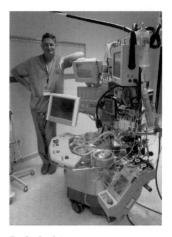

Perfusionist

Perfusionist: is a technician who looks after the heart/lung bypass machine during an open heart operation.

Pharmacist: makes up all the medicine prescribed for your child by the doctors and is based in the hospital.

Physiotherapist: will encourage your child to expand the lungs and breathe properly after surgery and will also help him or her to get out of bed and move normally.

Play Leader: is there to entertain your child and through play help him or her to understand what the doctors and nurses are doing and prepare your child for the operation.

Psychologist: can help children overcome needle phobia or other problems they may have with hospital admission and treatment.

Radiographer: is the person who takes x-ray pictures of your child's chest either in the x-ray department or with a portable machine on PICU or the ward.

Registrars and House Officers: cardiologists and surgeons have a team of doctors to help out with investigations and procedures. The most senior of these is the Registrar, and the juniors are the House Doctors. You may find that you see the registrar instead of the cardiologist or surgeon from time to time.

Social worker: you can discuss social or financial problems with a social worker who will be able to help you find the best way to deal with them.

Sonographer: is the person trained to carry out echos on your child.

Staff Nurse: a trained nurse who will look after your child while he or she is in hospital.

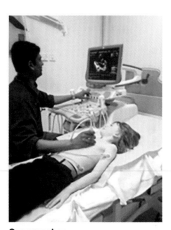

Student Doctor: most children's specialist heart hospitals are part of a teaching hospital. This means that Student Doctors may be present during the ward round or during tests and procedures. If you object to students being present, tell the senior member of staff present.

Student Nurse: is there to learn, gain experience and to carry out nursing and is supervised by the Staff Nurses and Sisters or Charge Nurses.

Sonographer

Theatre Sisters, Charge Nurses and Staff Nurses:
these nurses assist the surgeons while they operate on your child.

Ward Receptionist: this is the person who often answers the telephone, helps the doctors and nurses with a great deal of the paperwork necessary on the ward.

Ward Sister (female) or Charge Nurse (male): is responsible for the running of the ward and the nurses working in it.

Ward Cleaner: is the person who cleans the ward – try to keep the floor around your child's bed clear so that they can do the important job of keeping infection away.

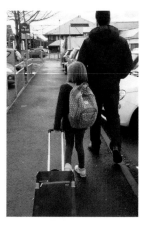

Being admitted to hospital

If the time comes when your child needs to be admitted to a hospital for surgery or a catheter procedure it is best to be as well prepared as possible, so that you in your in turn can help your child.

You may have already been in hospital when your child was a baby, so know a little of what to expect. If not, it can be intimidating to see all the machinery with flickering lights and alarms going off, and nurses and doctors rushing round, children attached to strange equipment, tubes and wires everywhere and babies hardly visible amongst it all! And if you have been in before, you may be overcome by the same emotions you had when your child was admitted, perhaps as an emergency.

Off to hospital

Take any opportunity, such as a preadmissions appointment, to familiarise with all those aspects of life in hospital – how much should you bring in? Can you wash your, or your child's, clothes? Can you use your mobile? Where will you be staying? Can other children stay overnight? What care can you give your child on the ward – eg toileting, feeding, washing?

By this time you will have had a chance to find out what is wrong with your child's heart and what an operation involves. If you have not been able to do so and your own GP has not been able to help (in such a specialised subject, not every doctor will know about all the recent advances in heart surgery) get in touch with your child's Named Nurse or your child's cardiologist. Remember you need to understand and agree with what is happening before you can give informed consent.

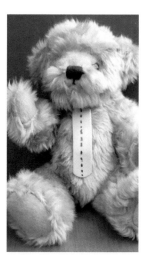

Your local parents' support group will also be able to help you by introducing you to a parent whose child has had a similar heart surgery or procedure. **See Chapter 13 Sources of help and support** for where to find more information.

Preparing your child

If your child is old enough, talk about going into hospital. The older your child, the longer he or she needs to get used to the idea. If he or she has been in hospital before remember together all the nice things about the stay and play out these situations with his or her teddy. Stick a plaster on teddy's leg or chest for example. Buy a toy stethoscope and listen to teddy's chest 'like the doctors and nurses did'. Encourage play about staying in hospital – if your child is older than four, Playmobil have sets of play people and hospital equipment including the hospital room, and the operating theatre – you might find these very useful in getting your child to talk about their fears, and to reassure them. Younger children may like to use drawings, or pictures from books published by heart groups.

Of course you will say that the hospital is to help the child feel better. It is a difficulty that we as parents face that often our children don't remember ever feeling well, so have nothing they can look forward to.

In this case you could say that the hospital will help to stop him or her from getting ill. Older children can have as much of an explanation about the heart condition and how it can be helped or fixed as suits their understanding. Don't overpromise – for example, recovery after a big operation may be slow, or if your child is on an anticoagulant after surgery, he or she may be more limited in choice of sports than before.

Contact the ward and ask to speak to the play specialist before admission if you need help in preparing your child. You will want to ask to see the psychologist if your child has developed a needle phobia or any major problem which is likely to interfere with treatment. You will need to take advice if your child has been diagnosed with, or is suspected of having, Autism or Aspergers.

Answer all questions as honestly as you can – if you don't know the answer, encourage your child to ask his or her special nurse, or the Play Specialist when you get to the hospital. The biggest reassurance you can offer is that you will be nearby, even when you are out of sight, and you will know what is happening to your child all the time.

A word of warning about admissions – it is not unusual for a surgery to be postponed because of shortages of intensive care beds, or infection on the ward, or your own child contracting untimely chicken pox. You will be asked to ring and let the hospital know if your child develops symptoms of infection – cough, cold, temperature, vomiting or diarrhea – in the run up to the admission date. You will need to call the day before admission to check that the bed is still available. So bear it in mind when planning the day when you and your child travel off to hospital – it will **probably** be the big day. If your child's admission is cancelled for a non-clinical reason (he or she is well enough for surgery) you should be offered another binding date for surgery within 28 days.

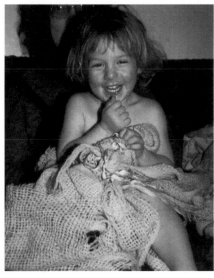

Comforter - well worn favourite.

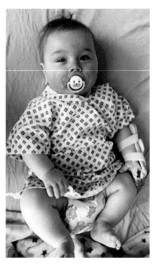
Don't forget my dummy

What to take

Better to tell your child he or she can choose just one favourite toy to take, and tuck a few others away in your bag, rather than invite a battle over the contents of the bedroom being packed. Don't worry if the comforter or toy is the well worn favourite which would look more at home in a rubbish bin than a hospital bed – it is nothing the hospital staff won't have seen before! But do label these with your child's name: they are easily mislaid.

With younger children, the familiar story book read a hundred times already may be more of a comfort than an interesting new book, so take both. Check that the must-have DVD is available on the ward and how you can arrange to secure it - or if you can, bring your own child's favourites. If you take musical toys, beware – you (and hospital neighbours) may have to listen to it many thousands of times, day and night.

More practically, take in any special bottles or feeding cups and any particular dietary preparation your child has been prescribed. Apart from when children go into the operating theatre, intensive care or catheter lab they should be able to wear their own clothes - choose comfortable and fairly cool day and night-time clothes – the ward will be kept warm – with opening down the front to help give access to the chest, a small supply of nappies if used, toiletries and any mobility aids, and medicines your child is taking whether prescribed or alternative. Older children will want to take their own tablets and mobiles. Do check if this is OK with the ward first, and remember to warn your child about the chances of losing things in such a public space.

Your child's paperwork includes the admission letter, GP details and health record. You yourself will need comfortable, crushable, cool clothes, toiletries, your own medication (you will not be able to get this from the hospital), cash and cards - which you will need to keep on your own person at all times – and a list of telephone numbers in case your mobile isn't working. Remember anything that is of spiritual importance to you and your child.

You may want to take reading material, and if you have an older child who will not need your undivided attention, you may have time to settle down with your book, Kindle or etc. However, assume that this is unlikely to be the case and take something you can occupy yourself with for short periods of time – magazines, Sudoku, crosswords. Do not take precious items with you. Keep expensive important items on your person – such as camera, watch, jewelry, bank card. Unthinkable as it may seem, people exist who would take advantage of your preoccupation with your sick child to steal from you.

Before setting off to the hospital you should get a leaflet telling you all about the facilities, where you can stay, whether you will have internet access, transport and parking, and local shopping. If you haven't seen this, you may be able to find details on line, or call the hospital number and ask for the information. If you have a disabled parking badge, check to see if this can be used in hospital parking areas.

On the ward

When you are welcomed on the ward you should be given information about hygiene, to keep your child and all other patients safe. The basic requirements are that you keep your hands clean and report any infection that you or visitors or people you are in close contact have. And hospitals may have their own rules to prevent the spread of infection - you may have to cover your shoes, or leave your coat or jacket outside the ward for example.

You should be told the names of your child's consultant, and nurse for that day. When you are welcomed onto the ward, you will need to pass the child's medicines and foods over for safe keeping, and a nurse will take down information as to your child's eating and sleeping patterns, likes and dislikes, special words for toileting or toys. Your child will be given an identity bracelet with name and hospital number – this must be checked by anyone who is involved in treating him or her. Check before taking your child to the toilet - samples may need to be measured, or nappies weighed before you can dispose of them.

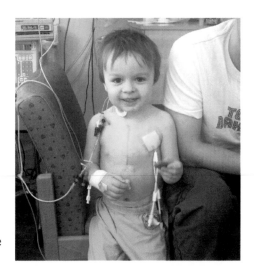

If you have other children with you, they are your responsibility – you must arrange for their care and meals, and make sure they behave in a way that is acceptable on the ward (this may not be the normal behaviour of healthy active noisy toddlers, so be prepared to take them off the ward). The hospital staff will not be able to babysit. All this is very hard, but there are times when the needs of others just cannot be accommodated.

Your child's bed area will have some limited storage space, and a bed or chair for you to stay nearby. You will be asked to observe hygiene rules – using gel to clean your hands when coming onto the ward, for example.

A nurse or doctor will examine your child and go through the medical history. If your child hasn't had a preadmission day for tests beforehand, he or she or she will be checked for infections, and have tests, such as an echo, x-ray and blood taken, to make sure all is well before surgery, and to give the doctors information on which to base post-operative treatment.

When blood is taken, a local anesthetic in the form of a cream is put on the skin so that there is no pain. Some heart children have very difficult veins to get into and this can be as distressing to the parent as to the child, but in most cases a cannula – a tube – will be put in your child's arm and kept there, so that blood can be taken without needing to go through all that again. If a urine specimen is needed and your child is not potty-trained, a plastic bag is attached to the genital area to catch the urine.

The surgeon who will be performing the operation should be visiting you and your child to talk through the operation and answer any questions you have. In earlier discussions you should both have been given enough information to feel that you know what will happen, why, when, and how. This should have included any complications that may happen as a result of the surgery and your child's chances of making a full recovery, but do check any aspect of the whole process you do not feel wholly informed about. Often children want to know where the scar will be, and what it will look like. After this you will be asked to sign the consent form.

The anesthetist will usually come to talk to you, check your child's mouth for loose teeth which could come out while the child is unconscious, and discuss any allergies or breathing problems, such as asthma, your child has.

A nurse will take you to get to know the Pediatric Intensive Care Unit (PICU): unless it is a straightforward operation, when he or she may be returned to the High Dependency Unit (HDU) or a ward, this is where your child will be taken after surgery. You will probably be able to see another child in this room with all the equipment attached. You may want to take your child to see PICU, but of course when sedated in a cot the view will be very different, and you will want to be sure he or she will not be upset by the sight of silent children apparently restrained and in pain. You could just say that he or she will be in a special room, where there will be doctors and nurses with machines to help in every way, even to breathe. He or she will not be able to talk, but will hear people talking and be able to mouth words and the nurses will understand. Remind your child that you will be nearby all the time (if this is so).

Boys may be upset to find that they have a line going into the penis – and either a son or a daughter may be alarmed at not being able to use a toilet, so explain in the words they understand that urine will be taken away so they will not be wetting the bed. Another thing you should say is that at first he or she may not be able to have anything to drink. His or her mouth will feel very dry, but the nurses will wet the mouth to make it feel better, with a little sponge dipped in water.

Back on the ward, at some point when you need to leave your child – you may want to take your bags to store them if you are staying in a room nearby, for example –

mention to the staff that you are going, and if you are in a cubicle area bring the child to the play area, where an eye can be kept on him or her. The same applies when you need to leave the ward to get a drink or have a meal. Do not take your child off the ward unless you have been told specifically that you can. Remember to put the cotsides up whenever you leave your child's side.

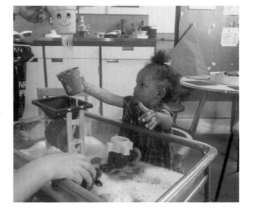

Run up to surgery

You will be told when food or drink will be stopped some hours before the operation. If your child is early on the operating list, he or she may be woken during the night to have a last drink. About one hour before going to theatre, he or she will be given premedication – usually a liquid medicine which will make him or her sleepy.

A porter will come to take your child and medical records to the anesthetic room. In most cases you can accompany the child, and even carry a small child or baby yourself. It is understandable that your own rising levels of fear and emotional turmoil make it difficult to keep a child calm as you approach the wished for but dreaded event. But a confident smile, words of reassurance that soon after the special sleep you will see your child again, and a quick kiss, will be of far more help to your son or daughter than the terrifying sight of a distressed parent.

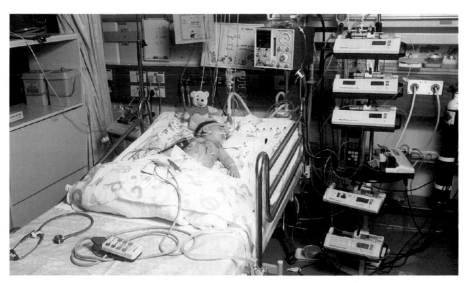

Your child will return to the Intensive Care Unit immediately after the operation.

When you leave your child, be kind to yourself and take a few minutes to recover. Many mothers and fathers find that they are overwhelmed by their feelings at this time, so you may want to give yourself permission to let pent up emotion break out.

Waiting

The next few hours will probably seem the longest of your life. If the weather is fine, it is a good idea for you to go out for a walk, or to go shopping, or to visit a museum: anything, in fact, to occupy you physically and while away the time, although your thoughts may well stay firmly in the hospital. You will be given an approximate time to come back to the hospital and can keep in touch with your mobile.

An open heart surgery can take anything from three to six hours, sometimes longer, and other operations about two to four hours, but delays are frequent – so do not be over anxious. A delay does not mean that anything has gone wrong. The staff know how you are feeling and will try to give you information from time to time.

Intensive Care Unit

When your child is ready, a bed which has been specially prepared is taken to the theatre and he or she is transferred straight onto it from the theatre operating table. The bed is then wheeled back to the ICU, and your child is attached to all the necessary equipment. He or she may then have his or her chest x-rayed and an echo. After all this you should be allowed to visit.

If the hospital treats adults as well as children, the ICU may be called a PICU – for Pediatric Intensive Care Unit. Your first visit to the PICU with its array of high technology equipment can be awe-inspiring and it is unlikely that you will be able to take it all in. Ask about anything you do not understand. Because a bypass machine is used during open heart surgery, the artificial circulation of blood takes a toll on the body systems. The lungs are collapsed and have to reinflate, the child needs to learn to breathe again for him or herself, and the fluids in the body need to be balanced. The wounds both internally and externally must heal, and of course the heart, which was stopped for a time, has to learn its rhythm again. We describe here what most children will need in the way of support after open heart surgery, while they recover.

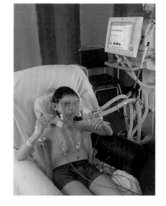

Your child's breathing is done by a machine called a ventilator. He or she will have a tube down the nose or mouth into the windpipe. This allows for the passage of air and oxygen from the ventilator to and from the lungs. To prevent it being dislodged, the ventilator tube may be attached with a band of strapping to your child's forehead. This tube is attached to a longer length of tubing which in turn is connected to the ventilator itself – a small machine standing beside the bed.

When your child is able to breathe completely unaided, he or she will be nursed with an oxygen facemask – or through a tube fixed under the nose which feeds oxygen to each nostril. Moisture is added to the oxygen, to keep chest secretions loose and easier to cough up. There will be another tube down his or her nose into the stomach allowing secretions to drain out and so prevent him or her from being sick.

There may be a drip going into a vein on one side of your child's neck. This is so that he or she can be fed intravenously – that is into a vein. Both arms may be splinted so that they cannot be moved and dislodge the equipment. There will be further tubes into veins to provide a means of giving blood or other fluid, to measure his or her blood pressure and to give some drugs if necessary.

There will be a tube into an artery: this is so that arterial (red) blood can be easily obtained for the frequent checks that have to be made on the gas and chemical content of the blood, to make sure that all the body systems are functioning correctly. This saves your child having frequent needle pricks. It also means that the blood pressure can be measured constantly, so your child doesn't have to be disturbed by having a blood pressure cuff put round his or her arm or leg frequently.

The pressures, along with heart rate, electrical activity and other vital technical information, are constantly measured through all the various wires attached to your child, and are continuously shown on a monitor screen.

The operation scar will be either down the middle of the chest or under the arm, with a dressing over the wound. If your baby's heart has swollen as a result of the surgery it may not fit into the chest, so the breast bone cannot be closed up after the surgery. Alarming as this sounds, a dressing covers the wound and the heart recovers in a day or two, when your child will be taken back to theatre to have the wound closed.

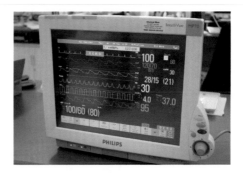

There will be one or two tubes coming out of his or her chest to drain off any fluid left in the chest cavity or around the heart. The amount is measured and a similar quantity of blood or other fluid is replaced. There are two pacing wires coming out of the chest which are usually rolled up in a little packet – they are there in case the natural pacing mechanism of the heart is temporarily affected by the surgery. If this happens, the wires are attached to an external machine which paces the heart and keeps it regular. Finally there is a tube which drains the bladder of all urine. This is measured to see how well the kidneys are working and what the child's fluid balance

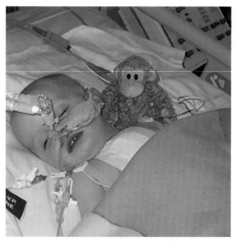

is. Remember that in PICU hygiene is even more important - this will certainly include hand cleaning and letting staff know about infections that you or anyone you or visitors may have been in contact with. In some hospitals you may be asked to leave your coat or jacket outside, and to wear an apron.

When you first come in to the PICU your child will probably be asleep, and will remain sedated for the first few hours.   Don't worry if he or she is awake, because if you ask later on, you will find that he or she will remember very little about this first day. Around this time you should get a report from the surgeon, or the surgeon's registrar, about how the operation went, and what was done. If your child was cyanosed (blue) before the operation it may come as something of a shock to see a pink-lipped infant where you expected to see your blue-tinged son or daughter. It is the first change that many parents notice.

There will be a nurse and a doctor (Intensivist) looking after your child all the time. You will be able to come and visit whenever you like but nobody will expect you to stay for long periods. You will probably be asked to check with a member of staff before entering PICU as there are very busy times, with doctors and nurses having to concentrate on the care of a number of children. Because of patient confidentiality, staff members will not give information about your child to people who telephone – if you cannot take the call yourself they will pass on a message and you could call back later. It is a very good idea to select a trusted friend or relative to whom you send frequent messages to pass on to others.

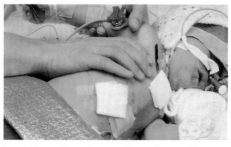

Physiotherapy is an important part of recovering.

Your child's nurse will be constantly checking on everything at least every fifteen minutes. Although the machines help the nurses and doctors a great deal, they cannot do the actual nursing!

You will quickly notice that the machines in the PICU keep up a chorus of bleeping noises and that from time to time, alarms appear to go off, adding to the stressful atmosphere. It is easy to be frightened by all this – or to misinterpret the information on the monitors if you are not medically trained. If in doubt, ask someone. The staff will be able to explain.

You will notice on occasions that the nurse will encourage your child to cough by applying suction to the tube in the windpipe, the nostrils and the mouth. This is done to prevent pooling of secretions in the lungs and to minimise the onset of chest infection. Chest physiotherapy will be given regularly by the physiotherapist. Intensive care nursing goes on throughout the night.

Don't feel that you need to stay with your child all the time – you should have a bed nearby. The day will have been mentally very exhausting for you, and you may find that you need several hours on a telephone to deal with the worries and concerns of your family.

If, for any reason, the doctors are worried, or there is anything they think you should know, they will contact you. Or, if you wake up during the night and want to know how your child is, all you have to do is dial the internal number of the ward and talk to the sister or staff nurse in charge.

When all is going well and tests are satisfactory the chest tubes and pacing wires will be removed. The ventilator will be gradually turned down so that your child has to make an effort to breathe by him or herself – once breathing is established the tube in the windpipe can be removed. Drinks are restricted, and you can help by keeping your child's mouth moistened. When he or she does start to drink, the amount of fluid given has to be limited at first because if he or she has too much, the kidneys may not be able to function properly. Therefore, you will be asked to measure all the fluid your child drinks.

Don't be too disappointed if your child seems to be taking longer than others to lose the tubes – it can take days or even weeks. The rate of progress varies from child to child depending on the severity of the heart defect and the sort of operation performed. Once most of the tubes have been removed your child will be move from the Intensive Care Unit to the ward, normally via the High Dependency Unit.

You will see that children are encouraged to sit out of bed and move around as soon as they are able. In a straightforward recovery it is not unknown for normal eating to be resumed within 24 hours of coming out of the operating theatre. More usually there will be a gradual return to normal eating – if your child had to be tube fed before surgery, you may find that he or she is now able to enjoy a bottle, or try solids for the first time. Gradually normal activity will be resumed, but you may notice that your child is tired, grumpy and miserable, and rather cross with you. This is a normal reaction and the older your child the more marked these 'post-op blues' tend to be. Encouraging your child to be involved with other children and playing on the ward can take the stress out of your relationship, which may have been very one-to-one over the previous week or so.

Sometimes the stitches closing the drain tube wounds and pacing wires won't be removed until your child is on the ward. By this point you may be starting to use the H word – home!

Going home

Although you may be given a probable day for going home – the discharge date – there is rarely absolute certainty. Some people have the delightful experience of being discharged earlier than expected, and an unfortunate minority will find they have to stay longer than they thought.

In some cases you may be advised that your home needs adaptations and extra equipment – a ramp for getting into the house, refrigeration and central heating for example, and these should be sorted out with the social services in your local council while your child is an inpatient.

Whatever your situation, plan your return home with the same attention as you planned going into hospital. Having anxiously searched out new friends to say goodbye to, it is all too easy to grab the medicines, the child and the luggage, and bundle everything into a hastily parked car, without carefully checking that you have all the information you need.

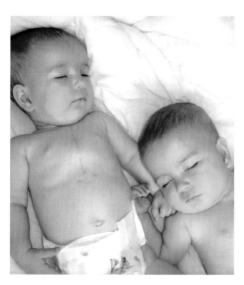

There will be a discharge plan for your child which should be discussed with you – this could be before the operation, so keep a note of anything you may need to ask after the operation.

Before you leave you should get a discharge leaflet, but make sure you have all the following information: Who to contact if you need advice? This could be the local hospital where your child is normally seen. There may be particular symptoms that you need to look out for. How to care for your child's wound – does it need to be cleaned or bathed? When should you approach your GP, health visitor, local children's ward, A&E, etc? Are there stitches that will need to be removed, or blood tests that need to be carried out? Do you need to arrange these yourself, or has your community team been notified? Ask for copies of letters to your GP or local pediatrician if they have not been given to you. If you have not been given a comprehensive hand-held record, ask when you will get one.

What medicines and special foods does your child need, how do these need to be given, and for how long? These should be given to you from the hospital pharmacy, and usually you will have to order follow-up supplies through your GP from your local pharmacist, so find out when the supply will run out and how long reordering will take –medicines sometimes have to be ordered in especially for your child. If your child uses oral syringes to take liquid medicines, make sure the hospital pharmacist prescribes them. In particular check when the next doses are needed after you leave the hospital.

If your child has feeding problems – how will you be put in touch with a local dietician? How will any special equipment such as NGTs be ordered and delivered?

You need to know what your child's new diagnosis is, and what the prognosis – the longer-term outlook – is. This should be spelled out in the letter to your GP, but you may need it translated into simpler English.

Ask about new or revised benefit claims, such as tax credit and DLA, and the time and place for your child's follow-up appointment. This could be at the PCU or at a clinic at a hospital near you attended by your child's consultant. If you cannot be given a date when you leave the hospital, get some idea of the optimum length of time – four to six weeks is the usual period – and ask how much warning of the date you will get.

You need to know what your child should be able to do and when – for example: starting or going back to school or nursery; swimming; playing competitive, contact or other games and sports; air travel and etc.

Lastly, make sure that the hospital has the correct contact details on the letters and records: GP details, child's name, hospital number, home address, telephone number should be checked so things don't go astray in future.

Your personal discharge plan will include what you and your child will wear to go home, how you are going to get there, and how you will manage feeding and medicine if this is a longer journey. If there is usually no one in during the day, you may want the heating turned on, beds made up and the shopping sorted out before you arrive. Discourage large welcome parties if you are the normal sort of parents who just want to settle the child, and any brothers and sisters, and then enjoy their own bathroom and own bed.

9. At home with the family

Bringing your new baby home from hospital is usually a time for celebration. But if he or she has been diagnosed as having a heart defect, or indeed has already undergone some investigation or surgery, the celebration may be marred with rather more than the usual anxiety. And bringing home an older child who has undergone heart surgery can also be a fraught experience.

Many parents talk of returning home and feeling very depressed. If their child has done well they feel guilty about this and cannot understand why they feel so low.

In reality, it is not easy taking back sole responsibility for your child's care, when in hospital there was always medical advice and support on tap. Also, for many weeks prior to and during hospitalisation, you will have been living on nervous energy with all other considerations not to do with your child having become irrelevant. The separation and splitting up of the family while your child was in hospital is one of the things that may cause problems when surgery is hopefully behind you. It takes quite an adjustment to get back into the routine of work, cooking, shopping and so on – all very mundane in comparison.

Home from hospital

Even a minor heart condition which has been repaired can cause a huge amount of anxiety, and you may be uncertain as to how to respond in terms of care for your child.

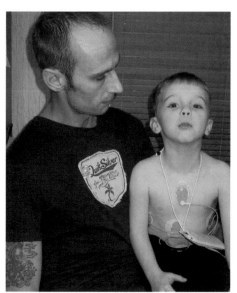

If this is your first, you should know that the healthiest of young babies have the ability to frighten us with their wobbly heads, snuffly noises, unspecified demands and generally alien behaviour. Be honest – have you woken a sleeping child to make sure he or she is OK? This sort of behaviour is particularly likely when, just out of hospital, you have spent four hours trying to get the child to sleep, and after an hour found the silence terrifying.

Problems with getting your child to sleep are not confined to those with heart conditions. But young children who are used to a hospital routine, may take longer to sort out. And if, as in many cases, your baby is a poor feeder, tires easily, falls asleep in the middle of his

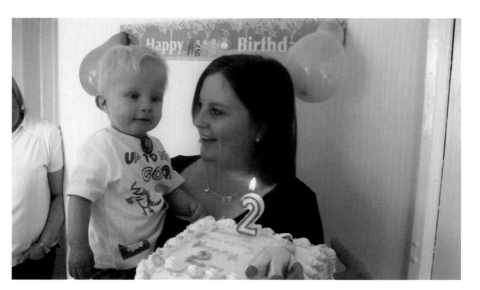

or her feed and then wakes up screaming an hour later, and maintains this pattern at night as well - you may well feel as though you are living in a waking nightmare.

Older children won't have a routine for a while, may be suffering from quite traumatic experiences, have pain or discomfort from recent surgery, or their new medicines may be causing nightmares. An older child is likely to be very clingy and may want to sleep in your bed, or to know where you are all the time, or display worrying symptoms every half hour or so.

Making times in your daily routine when your child can rest while pursuing normal activities such as listening to you read, or watching TV, can help to avoid those tantrums caused by sheer tiredness.

Keeping a diary of bedtime routines and night time activity can help to assure you that things are improving, but if things are not getting better, seek help from your GP, or health visitor, and remember to ask the pharmacist if your child is taking medicines that can cause sleep disturbance – there may be a better alternative.

Make sure of your support networks - let your GP know that you are home from hospital, and ask for the Health Visitor to call – don't wait for them to get in touch. If you feel concerned that something really is not right with your child, phone the number given to you before you were discharged, or the last ward you were on, and ask their advice.

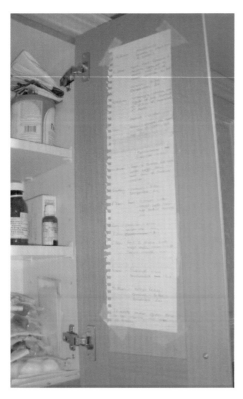

Prevention and precautions

Immunisation

You will want to check that your child's immunisation programme is kept up to date, and there may be additional protection recommended – bronchiolitis can be a particular threat to children with heart disorders. Ask your child's Named Nurse about extra immunisations and how safe they are. Nasal spray flu immunisation must not be given to children who are on an anticoagulant. If your child has allergies, remember to check they are on all his or her medical records. Making sure your older children are also immunised is important to minimise the risk of infection.

Medicines

Check with your local pharmacist before giving your child any over the counter medicine – for example even some teething gels cannot be used if your child is on an anticoagulant such as warfarin.

If your child is taking a small dose of aspirin, some doctors advise that you stop it if his or her temperature rises, so ask what you should do.

Teeth

If your child has a heart problem, an increase in bacteria getting into the blood stream could cause an infection of the heart called endocarditis. This is extremely rare. The risk is increased due to sluggish blood flow.

A small amount of bacteria get into our blood all the time, and they are destroyed by the immune system. But if

Echocardiogram showing 'vegetation' caused by endocarditis (arrowed).

116

the conditions in your child's mouth, such as a tooth abscess, allow a large number of bacteria to breed – we are talking millions here – and to get into the blood stream, the immune system may lose the battle to stop them settling on the lining of the heart and valves.

You need to limit the amount of sugar that gets into your child's mouth, and the length of time it stays there. Sugar is found in a lot of prepared food and drinks – not just sweets and biscuits. Avoid them whenever you can. After your child has sweet food or drink give plain water to rinse his or her mouth. Smaller children can swallow the water, larger children can spit it out. At the same time your child's diet should include the calcium that will help build up the strength of the enamel on their second teeth – found in milk, cheese and meat. Raw vegetables act as natural cleaners, and strengthen teeth as they are chewed, but remember that most fruit and even natural fruit drinks have sugar and acid.

If your child needs high calorie foods, butter, cream and yoghurt are better at increasing his or her weight than sugary foods, but in the real world there are children who will only eat half a chocolate button a day. Calories come first, so redouble your efforts to keep your child's mouth clean.

Ask the pediatric pharmacist at the hospital about getting sugar free medicines. Use oral syringes rather than teaspoons, as these allow the child to shoot the medicine beyond the part of the tongue that can taste how horrible it is, and away from the teeth. Swap to pills or tablets as soon as your child is old enough to swallow them.

Get rid of the plaque in your child's mouth. Clean teeth after meals. Small children who can't or won't have their teeth cleaned can chew on a soft rag, and rinse with clean water. However good your child may be with a toothbrush, clean his or her teeth yourself as well, until disclosing tablets (from your local pharmacist) show your child can do a thorough job.

And most important, take advice from your child's dentist: best when you first visit shortly after your child's birth or as soon thereafter as you can. Tell your dentist about the heart problem, and about the medicines your child is taking. It isn't just gum disease that can make your child liable to endocarditis. Piercings and tattoos can be particularly dangerous. Some children have heart defects that can be corrected and do not leave them vulnerable to endocarditis. If in doubt ask the cardiologist what is safe.

When to call the doctor

One of the major worries that parents have during the early months of caring for a heart baby is knowing whether or not he or she is unwell. As with any child one of the best indicators is going off food. A sudden change in behaviour pattern, such as an unusual degree of lethargy, or if the baby appears unusually pale or sweaty, can also be something to watch. Usually if a baby is taking food normally, there is no cause for concern.

Most GPs are very helpful and understand your anxieties, but readily admit that they generally have very few heart children to deal with and so do not always have the information you may be looking for. Many parents find the realisation that their GP's expertise is limited rather frightening. But although not a specialist on children's hearts, your GP knows a great deal about children's problems, the difference between being ill and well – and does have the responsibility for your child. You should not feel that you alone have to carry the burden of deciding when your child is ill.

Explain to your GP why you feel your child is unwell, and if you are requesting a visit at 2 am in the morning (isn't that always the time babies and children go from being unwell to ill?) instead of demanding that a doctor visit, take a deep breath, explain your concern and ask for advice. In most parts of the UK there is an out-of-hours number to call, NHS 111 in England and Wales, where you will have to go through a large number of questions first, so make every effort to be calm and rational.

Remember that if your child is showing signs of infection, a hospital ward is unlikely to welcome you visiting and infecting other children, so always call first.

If you have any worries that your child's heart condition could worsen suddenly while asleep, speak to the Named Nurse about monitoring. You may already have an alarm, but these are only good for hearing your child, not accounting for silences! Your Named Nurse or health visitor may suggest monitoring breathing – take advice before buying one of the devices on the market that can alert you to when your child's breathing cannot be detected. Some hospitals will provide you with monitoring equipment such as a pulse oximeter to measure oxygen saturations if your child has a condition which leaves him or her vulnerable to sudden deterioration.

Outpatient appointments

While your child is visiting the clinic, there will be a chance for you to voice any concern you are feeling at your child's condition. If you have several questions to ask, (and who hasn't?) write them down. Many parents complain of suffering a mental block when they are faced with a busy Outpatient Department and a doctor that they may not have seen before. Writing down in advance any questions you want to ask, helps overcome this problem.

Bringing up your child

If bringing up a healthy child is difficult enough, raising a child who has a heart condition inevitably presents us with problems we've not even thought of before, let alone had to deal with. We are continually beset with questions: to what extent should I enforce discipline? How much exertion can I allow? What about school, will he or she cope in a normal school environment?

It sometimes helps to turn the whole situation around and try to change the emphasis. Not 'here is a heart child, what can he or she do?' but 'here is an ordinary child who happens to have a heart condition, is there anything he or she cannot do?' Young children with heart conditions usually know their own physical limits, but you may be advised against him or her mixing with other children because of the risk of infection, or taking part in games at nursery when physical activity could cause an irregular heart rate.

Exercise

Older children with major heart problems may have to avoid over-strenuous exertion, or contact sports – those where collisions, buffeting and bruising are more likely - and will start to become aware that they cannot always keep up with their friends at school. Depending on your child's personality, this can cause a great deal of frustration. In either case, whether these are temporary or long-term problems, make sure you know why activities should be restricted, and which these are. Start thinking of some less physically demanding interest for your child: something at which he or she can be reasonably good at, as his or her ego may be taking a hammering in other areas. For children who are breathless, the advice is to stop the activity when they are too breathless to talk.

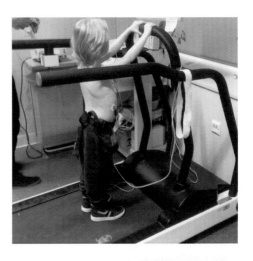

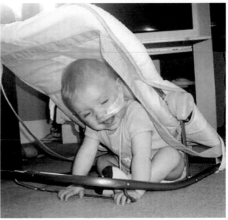

For the more physically able child, indoor basketball which uses a smaller area may be an alternative to football or netball when the weather is cold. Drama may serve as a useful outlet for some children. Giving your child a pet of his or her own to take care of is another possibility. The main thing to strive for, is as full and normal a life as possible and to try to avoid imposing unnecessary restraints. But bear in mind that most children need no restriction at all, and that limits placed on your child may no longer be necessary as time goes on. Check at least annually – your Named Nurse can help you.

Just a word about swimming – heart children who don't have a cyanotic heart condition, as well as those that do, can find swimming even in a heated pool causes them to become blue, shivery and very cold very quickly. Wetsuits, which do keep children warm, can be bought for all ages, and may be worth an investment,

119

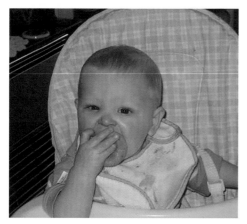

particularly if your child is limited in other activities and enjoys swimming. If your child has some forms of irregular heart beat (arrhythmia) swimming could be a danger to him or her. Check with the cardiologist.

Discipline

Discipline is basically a matter of teaching a child the rules by which he or she can live as an acceptable member of society. We are doing any child a disservice if we do not teach him or her these rules.

Many parents complain that their heart child is unusually irritable, tearful and lacking in concentration, particularly prior to surgery and for a time after surgery. Somehow, as parents, we have to try to walk a tightrope between accepting that there are times when our children find just carrying on as normal more than they can cope with, and teaching them that rudeness and temper tantrums are not acceptable modes of behaviour. And we have to persuade aunts and uncles and grandparents not to indulge bad behaviour because of their concern for the child.

Encouraging independence

As your child grows up try to give him or her the same responsibilities as any other young person in dealing with money, friends, and guarding their privacy. If the child will need ongoing treatment, make sure he or she has a planned transition to adult health care. When your child reaches 16, he or she becomes responsible for signing his or her or her own consent for medical treatment.

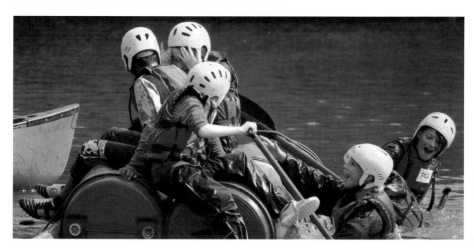

Even with a thoughtfully phased plan of increasing discussion and involvement over several years, it may not be easy to prepare your child for this situation. If he or she has never been encouraged to take responsibility for his or her or her condition, such a situation can be doubly traumatic for both of you. How you can help is to keep the lines of communication open at all costs. Let your son or daughter know that you are there to support him or her at all times, but don't try to make it better. You can't – and he or she knows this.

No matter how old your child is when surgery is needed, it is an incredibly difficult time. In our experience that feeling of helpless dread parents have does not go away as your child gets older. In many ways you may feel more helpless as your child becomes a young adult because you cannot shoulder his or her or her fears and anxieties. Your son or daughter has to take some steps alone and all you can do is to be, endlessly patient and prepared to listen if he or she wants to talk, or just to be there.

Brothers and sisters

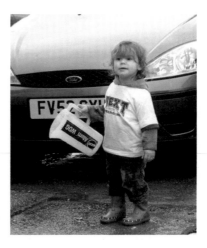

It is sometimes difficult for other children in your family to understand why their brother or sister may be the object of extra attention from grandparents and other relatives or friends. It is natural they may feel some resentment about this and they will find it easier to cope if they are helped to understand why it occurs.

This may be particularly the case when your baby is first diagnosed. An older brother or sister, if their baby brother or sister's illness is not explained, may feel that they are responsible for the illness because of naturally occurring jealousy at the new arrival. An older child of pre-school age may not understand any more than that the baby is ill but they can be encouraged to help with simple fetching and carrying tasks and be included in bathing and changing rituals. This will help children feel included and less anxious about the strain their parents are clearly under. When the baby is older, brothers and sisters need to be kept in touch with the situation.

If a spell in hospital is necessary, they will be better able to cope with the separation from both their parents and sibling if it has been talked over with them, so they know why it has to occur and exactly who will be looking after them while mum and/or dad is away at the hospital.

You may be very torn between looking after a child in hospital and a child at home, and have hard choices to make between caring for a toddler, or staying with a seven year old on the ward. Being with an older child at home over the period of important examinations or starting a new school, may have to be sacrificed if you are not to ignore the needs of a child undergoing necessary but painful experiences.

Advice from parents is to stay in regular touch with other children – if you are close enough to the hospital, having a slot perhaps in the late afternoon when you give other children exclusive attention can work. If you cannot see them at the hospital or at home, set a time of day when you will telephone just to speak to your children, so they know they haven't lost your interest and support.

You

A lot to cope with

Babies are remarkable barometers of their mothers' emotions, so the more anxious and worried you are feeling the more quickly your baby will home in and react adversely to your feelings, which in turn will obviously affect you. Coping with a convalescent child who clings to you, throws tantrums and is faddy about food, is not easy. Add your other children who may be feeling equally insecure as a result of the separation – and you have a lot to cope with!

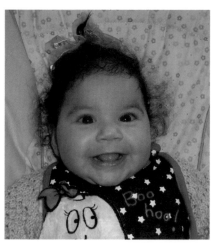

Break the cycle

One can very easily get into a seemingly endless cycle of worry and tension; it does help to be aware of this and try to break the cycle before it goes too far. During fraught periods when your own night time rest is disturbed, try to sleep when your child sleeps during the day, even if it's just fifteen minutes with your feet up.

If your baby will take breast milk or formula from a bottle, welcome offers to come and feed from time to time. Bonding with your child will not be undermined, and the anxiety you may feel will be dissipated for a while. If you feel things starting to get on top of you, try leaving your son or daughter with a trusted friend or relative, even if it is only for an hour and get out. Be very careful about turning down offers of help – no one can shop, cook, clean or look after your children the way you do, but reject support and it may not be offered when you really need it.

Do anything that makes a change from your normal routine so that you have the opportunity to distance yourself from your problems, even for a short time.

Anxiety is a strong emotion which creates energy: give it an outlet, such as a long walk, gardening or a spell in the gym.

Your relationship

Undoubtedly, having a child with a disability, and especially a life threatening condition, can create unexpected problems in parent relationships.

From the experience of other families, the biggest problem is that people react quite differently in the way that they deal with things. One parent may want to talk about the child and the child's health repeatedly, the other may want to avoid the subject as being too painful to deal with; one may search the internet tirelessly for information about the condition, the other may cling to the most comforting diagnosis and prognosis they can remember. Often one will try to withdraw emotionally a little, in an attempt to distance themselves from distress, another will try to anticipate the worst scenario by rehearsing it constantly to avoid the shock should it happen. It is hardly surprising that two people with such differing approaches can offend and hurt each other.

Another difficulty can arise when one partner blames the other for a condition: perhaps a father has followed an unhealthy lifestyle prior to the conception, perhaps the mother drank during the pregnancy. Inlaws have been known to join in the blame game, to the detriment of all involved.

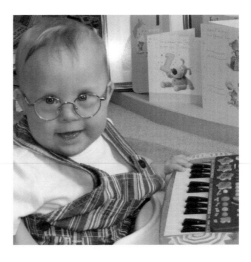

Exhaustion, financial worries, fear – not many people can support their partner at a time when they are experiencing looking after a sick child round the clock, taken a reduction in income, and living in constant fear for their child's wellbeing.

We do not have the answers – but by being aware that these problems may occur, that they may exist over a short period of time, and tolerating what may appear to be selfishness may get you through. If you cannot discuss how you are feeling with a discreet friend, use a helpline, one of the many closed (private) facebook groups online, or a support group where you can remain anonymous.

Your parents

Your own parents will probably be as anxious about you as you are about your child. This can make it a really difficult relationship, especially when you are the one with the knowledge and expertise about your child's condition, and don't need the advice you would perhaps normally seek.

Let parents know how they can help – for example, with financial support, as burdens often come when caring for your child destroys employment and career opportunities, or a commitment to care for other children when you have medical appointments.

Many have found comfort in being able to telephone regularly to someone who is concerned about the whole family, not just the child with the heart condition.

Other people

Some people who have never had a sick child, find it very difficult to understand what a strain it can be. It is very difficult to explain the sense of isolation one can feel when faced with the never-ending questions entailed in bringing up a heart baby. Why isn't he or she putting on weight? What will they say at the next hospital appointment? Is it normal for him to be late sitting up, crawling, walking? Does he or she seem more breathless, bluer than usual? What does the future look like?

It seems impossible sometimes to find someone willing to listen to your anxieties for as long as you want to voice them. Friends may expect you to react in a certain way, or they may react in a way you find difficult to accept. You may mention to a friend that you are worried about some aspect of your baby's condition, to have that friend reply that her 'non heart' baby is 'just the same'.

If you are looking for a sounding board at that particular time, this quite harmless reply may be reassuring or may be quite incredibly irritating. Other mothers wonder what to say to well-meaning strangers who look at their blue-tinged children and ask if they are wrapped up warmly enough.

Many parents have found joining a support group helps to put things in perspective. If you are feeling particularly anxious about how your baby will cope as he or she grows up, seeing another child with an equally severe problem coping well may help ease your fears and encourage you to feel more optimistic about the future. **See Chapter 13 Sources of help and support.**

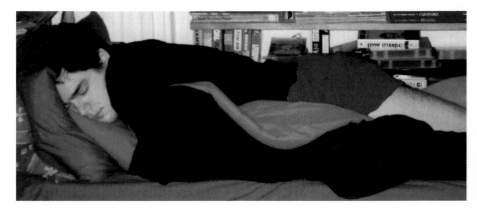

It can be difficult to fully support your son or daughter in taking over what, until now, has been your role for ensuring their best care, especially if this has been a large part of your life. And it is the experience of some parents that their adolescent has no inclination to take responsibility for themselves.

But by the age of 12, if your son or daughter has long-term treatment in their care plan, he or she will be set on the pathway to adult health care – you may hear this referred to as 'transition'. This can be a trying time, especially if your child has special needs. It will involve you making efforts to include him or her in understanding the heart condition, managing their own appointments and treatment schedules, and able to make the best use of the transition nurse, so that their opinions and feelings are heard and considered.

Many of us have found it hugely comforting to retain links with other parents who have seen their child to adulthood, where you can share private anxieties without compromising your son or daughter's privacy, and share your own valuable advice and insights.

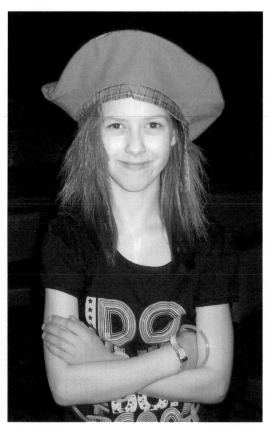

And finally

So to sum up, there will be times when you will feel as if no one understands your problems at all. Do not cut people out of your life because they appear to be out of sympathy with you at a particular time. The support of others will become more important to you as your child grows, so try not to become so wrapped up in his or her problems that you have no room for anyone else.

Try to maintain some outside interests. Don't ask too much of yourself and your partner – and do ask for help and advice if you are worried about anything. And remember that your child is his or her own person, who will want not just your love and concern, but your respect for their independent being.

10. Finances and work

Information here relates to England – benefits and support are largely similar but have some differences in Northern Ireland, Scotland, and Wales.

Citizen Advice Bureau has websites for all four parts of the UK which can give you accurate and up-to-date benefit information.

Having a child is expensive – this will not be news to you. And if you are faced with having a child with a health problem, there are inevitably extra calls on the family finances.

Take a child with a comparatively minor health problem – one which just needs watching to see if it will correct itself, such as a VSD which may close over time, but is accompanied by feeding difficulties – plans to return to work after the birth may be disrupted entirely, as feeding regimes and medical appointments take over for the first months or years.

There may be trusted child care and support available, and for some parents this will work out for them. But there is an emotional dimension to discovering a child's heart condition – one that can interfere with our reasoning processes and focus. So there may be a longer period of living on one less wage than you can have anticipated. Returning to work after a lengthy period away may be harder than you expect – a workplace may be unfamiliar and relationships difficult to re-establish, and a reduction in earning potential may result.

So over the period of time, at least to the point where your child's health status can be considered 'normal', and you can re-establish a normal working pattern, you may need extra support for your family finances.

Disability Living Allowance

If your child's heart condition and any other health problems mean that he or she needs a lot of extra care, there will be a benefit to help with the additional costs: Disability Living Allowance (DLA). Remember that eligibility for DLA is based on how much care your child needs above and beyond that of a child of a similar age, and not whether or not he or she has a heart condition.

To get DLA your child needs to be eligible: he or she must have had the need for extra care for three months or more, (unless sadly he or she is not expected to live longer than six months, when DLA can be claimed under Special Rules).

There are two components of DLA – Care and Mobility. Children can only get the higher rate of Mobility from the age of three, and from the age of five for the lower rate. DLA for Care can be awarded at either a low, medium or high rate.

DLA is not an easy benefit to get, but that doesn't mean that you shouldn't apply for it.

When applying for DLA for your child, you need to bear in mind that the person looking at your claim knows nothing about heart disease in children. All young children need lots of care so it is sometimes difficult to demonstrate that your child needs more. They will not understand how heart failure can undermine a child's abilities to participate in normal activities, and can create a need for extra calorific food and a warm environment. They don't know if your child's heart disease or a diagnosed or undiagnosed syndrome has caused slow growth, agonising pains in the limbs overnight, problems with hypermobility, bowel problems, learning difficulties, or allergies. They don't know if or why your child has behavioural problems, night terrors, feeding difficulties, lapses of consciousness or asthma. You will have to say if your child had a period of hypoxia or stroke, has no bladder control, and a medicine regime that demands hours of your time.

You don't have to say why your child has a condition eg reflux, or incontinence – because the reason may not have been diagnosed – but how the condition affects him or her and the amount of care you need to give because of it.

If you are awarded any DLA for Care for your child you will be able to get a top-up on any tax credit you are entitled to, and if your child is awarded DLA High Care rate an even greater child tax award could be paid. DLA may also affect housing benefit should you be in socially rented housing.

If your child is awarded DLA at Medium or High Rate Care and you choose to stay home with your child (or work part time up to a set earnings limit) and meet the criteria, then you may also be entitled to claim a carer's benefit for yourself, Carers Allowance. Having a child with a disability in receipt of DLA can exempt you from the 'benefit cap', and could entitle you to free child care. An award for mobility can be converted to a suitable car to help transport your child.

You can see the forms online at www.gov.uk/disability-living-allowance-children. Before you start to deal with them, contact the DLA Disability Living Allowance on 0345 712 3456. You can get a printed copy of the form and advice on completion, but most important, establish a date for your claim. If it is successful it will be paid back to the date you made that call. If at first you do not get awarded DLA you will need to put in for a Mandatory Reconsideration before you can go to Appeal. Take advice before doing this to give yourself the best chance of success.

You must tell the Department for Work and Pensions (DWP) if your child's care or mobility needs change while they're still getting DLA. You'll be invited to claim PIP if this happens.

DLA is only paid if your child is aged under 16 – once 16 he or she is considered to be adult and must claim the Personal Independence Payment in his or her own right.

Personal Independence Payment (PIP)

Young people getting Disability Living Allowance (DLA), will be invited to claim PIP when their DLA ends or when they reach the age of 16. PIP has replaced DLA for new claimants aged 16 to 64.

If your child receives DLA and is approaching the sixteenth birthday, the Department of Work and Pensions will write to you to ask whether the young person will need an appointee from age 16: that is to say, whether he or she can represent him or herself. Then, at age 16 a letter will be sent inviting the young person or the appointee to claim PIP. DLA payments will continue (even if it was due to expire) while the PIP claim is being processed.

Remember that a young person will not be automatically transferred from DLA to PIP, so call the Disability Centre Tel: 0345 712 3456 if your child's sixteenth birthday is in less than four weeks and you haven't received a letter.

PIP is difficult to claim successfully – make sure your young person knows where to get help and advice before sending off the forms.

Carers Allowance

If your son or daughter gets Disability Living Allowance (DLA) or Personal Independence Payment (PIP) at the middle or highest care rate, and you spend at least 35 hours a week looking after them, you may be able to claim Carers Allowance. Take advice before claiming – it is taxable and can reduce your or your child's benefits

Getting up to date advice on benefits is important

- There is up-to-date guidance on the Citizens Advice Bureau Website – www.adviceguide.org.uk. Information about benefits including hints and tips on how to make a successful claim can also be found on the many support groups' websites and facebook pages. If your support group is for your child's particular syndrome or heart condition, you will probably be able to get expert help from that source.
- The best way to establishing what state benefits you personally may be able to get is to use Turn2Us facility. Turn2Us is a national charity which allows you to find what financial help is available in your situation.
- Contact a Family (helpline 0808 808 3555) can give you up-to-date guidance. You will also find help with other services available to families with your problems – SENDirect is a service Contact a Family run online, and lists by your area resources such as emergency child-minding, respite care and holidays.
- If you are unable to get online to see websites at home, and you are able to get out, a Citizens Advice Bureau, local library or jobcentre should be able to get you access.

Extra expenses

You may find that is impossible to stretch finances for some of the expenses that arise – a broken down washing machine needs to be replaced, a car seat is too small....
There are often local charities throughout the country that can help out: your local authority is always a good place to start – ask for Welfare Advice – or try a local library.

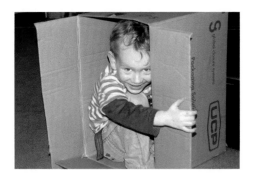

- Family Fund (www.familyfund.org.uk tel 01904 621115) will look at any grant request that relates to the needs of a disabled or seriously ill child, young person and their family, such as providing furniture, car seats, clothing, bedding, washing machine, sensory toys, computers or tablets, a family break, or something to help with college for 16 and 17 year olds.
- React (www.reactcharity.org tel 020 8940 2575) provides basic essential needs in families where a child has terminal or life-limiting illness, such as specialist or medical equipment (unavailable through your Health Authority), educational equipment (to aid your child's development when at home or in hospital), domestic equipment (household items which contribute to your child's comfort or quality of life), hospital expenses (travel, food or related costs) and can offer holidays for the family.
- SSAFA the Armed Forces charity helps all serving members and former members of all ranks of the Armed Forces and their families. Call 0800 731 4880 to find out what support is available.
- Children's Heart Federation (www.chfed.org.uk tel 0808 808 5000) can make a grant available for hospital travel and other exceptional expenses. If your child is on warfarin and you have to travel frequently to a clinic for INR tests, CHF may be able to help if you cannot get a home testing device from your GP.
- Many of the national, local and condition specific support groups provide caravan holidays, help with medical equipment, trips out during those expensive summer holidays, as well as general support and advice. Again Contact a Family (0808 808 3555) can help you find schemes that meet your need.

Working

Some of the best support, both financially and for your morale, is being in paid employment. It is ironic that just when you need an income to support a family, a disabled child can cause parents' career prospects to nosedive.

You are probably only too well aware of the problems: finding suitable care for your child, finding employment that offers the hours you can work, having flexibility for medical appointments and periods in hospital, earning enough to cover expenses and loss of benefit income, and getting up to speed with new working practices, let alone finding and competing for a job.

Overcoming the emotional ties to a child whose life has been threatened by illness can be the hardest thing of all, and demands of caring can be exhausting. The advantages can be that you keep your hand in at a chosen career, raise your income, reassert your identity, have something else to think about, and perhaps reduce the isolation that often comes with the full-time role of carer.

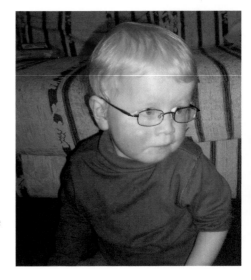

Everyone's circumstances are different: for some people sharing caring and working between two parents can be the answer, one working full-time and one part-time can release enough hours, self-employment or working from home may be a possibility.

Certainly employers are encouraged to pursue family-friendly policies, and your situation will not be new to most of them.

- To get a handle on whether working is an option for you, get in touch with Contact a Family helpline - tel 0808 808 3555 – and ask if you would be better off financially in work and what support you can expect.
- There is a Working Families Helpline, that can help with employment rights and law: www.workingfamilies.org.uk, tel 0800 013 0313.

11. Childcare and education

When a baby enters your life you expect to spend most of your time caring for him or her, perhaps to make arrangements for childcare when returning to work, and later to organising the best educational experience you can. But depending on your heart child's health and abilities, deciding on his or her care and education inside and outside of the home can be something of a problem. In this chapter we are looking at what difficulties you may face, and sources of information and advice that can help you through them.

Care in your home

If you know your child has special needs from before birth or from a very young age, you may want to contact Portage. If this organisation is operating in your area a home visitor will help you with the skills and confidence you need, no matter what your child's difficulties are.

As well as the usual love and care, catering for a heart child's needs may take up long periods of time. Sometimes a heart child may have severe reflux, or food aversion, and need medication or even tube feeding to deal with it. On top of this, you may be busy with medical appointments, hospital stays, and still need to parent other children.

For some families,employing a nanny privately can be the answer – either someone who lives in your home, or comes in by the day.

This arrangement has some advantages – your child's specific needs can be met, and he or she can be cared for when too unwell to go out for example. Look carefully at how you select the nanny – perhaps through a Nanny agency which carries out the checks and remains the employer, or finding someone you employ directly yourself. If you become the employer, you will need to pay tax and national insurance, sick pay and have other legal responsibilities. Look carefully at the costs and how long and for how many hours you will expect to employ a nanny for – you may want your child to socialise with others at a nursery as he or she gets older for example.

Unlike other childcare providers, nannies are not registered by the local authority, nor are they inspected by Ofsted, but nannies in England can register on the Ofsted Childcare Register if they fulfil training requirements and there are equivalent arrangements in Northern Ireland, Scotland and Wales.

Being a person's employer as well as sharing your children with him or her (remember the mannies as well as the nannies) can be difficult – if you are the kind of person who finds it difficult to accept other people feeding or playing with your children, or enjoying their affection, a nanny is probably not for you.

Preschool care

Most children with heart conditions will be able to go to the same childminders, playgroups, nurseries and schools as their brothers and sisters. But you, like most parents, will want to be sure that while your child is safe, he or she will enjoy the opportunities open to all children. Maybe your child needs extra naps at a day nursery, finds cold weather a struggle, needs extra snacks to keep up their weight, for example. They may not qualify as disabled or having special educational needs, but you will have to make sure the people looking after your child are kept up to speed with your child's needs, and your aim will be for your child to be treated as normally as possible.

There are new standards for under-fives called Early Years Foundation Stage Framework (EYFS). All early years providers must meet these standards to ensure that children learn and develop well – these are all (not just local authority) school leaders and staff, nurseries, private nursery schools, childminders, preschools and playgroups. Your local authority should have a Special Educational Needs Coordinator (SENCO) in the Early Years team who can help you with extra support in pre-school settings and can explain what services you can expect locally. These will include childcare that is able to support your child's Special Educational Needs and Disabilities (SEND). All childcare providers should make sure your child has the same play and learning opportunities as other children and should not charge you more for providing extra support.

It will be worth speaking to your Family Information Service, which can provide details of all the registered childcare providers in your area, as well as information on flexible working and benefits – this is also based in your local authority.

Once you have selected a child care provider – say a child minder or nursery – you should complete a care plan. Usually you will be given a form to complete, but do not be afraid to add to it if it does not cover all aspects of your child's possible needs. The staff are less likely to understand the possible consequences of your child's heart condition than more common health conditions in children, so include any problems to look out for eg needing to be toileted frequently because taking diuretics, no rough play as on aspirin or warfarin, avoiding hitting in the chest, rest place for periods of tiredness, extra time for eating.

Some unfortunate blue (cyanosed) children have been wrapped in blankets and generally overheated - remind the carers how to know if he or she is cold. Provide an explanation for your child's scars, and how the child feels about them (some children will insist on raising their top to show their scar to any passing adult, others will refuse to look at it or acknowledge it). If your child has a pacemaker, you will need to say that a defibrillator (for restarting the heart) must not be used in the unlikely event that your child loses consciousness. (We find that staff most often ask what to do if the child loses consciousness – the same as such an episode in another child – call an ambulance you might think!)

Remember to include any other problems your child has, such as allergies which are not related to the heart condition – if the staff only focus on the heart condition they may overlook these. A MedicAlert bracelet alerts people to your child's hidden conditions, and provides a link to medical records available 24/7.

This care plan should be updated when anything changes and renewed every half-term – hopefully to remove some of the problems which have now disappeared and to make sure contact numbers are up-to-date, but also to bring it to the attention of staff again.

Your child's nursery, pre-school or childminder will write an Early Years Foundation Stage profile when he or she moves into a reception class. This will give details about your child's strengths, talents and likes, as well as any additional support that he or she has needed.

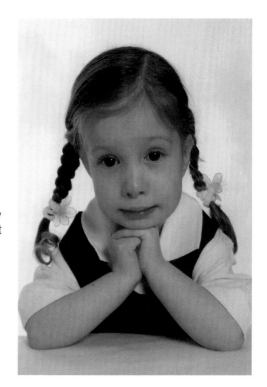

Education Health Care (EHC) Plan

If you believe your child is going to need support over and above that available from childcare providers, you can ask for an EHC assessment.

A child has special educational needs (SEN) if he or she has much more difficulty learning than others of the same age, or a disability that makes it hard to benefit from the facilities generally available in local schools, or if this is likely to be so, once he or she reaches school age.

If your child has SEN **and** it may be necessary for special educational provision to be made for him or her, you can ask the local authority for an EHC assessment.
Your child care provider can also ask for an assessment, as can a school or college or the child themselves when they are older.

Before agreeing the content of the request to the local authority, talk to people who know about your child's problems or potential problems – if your child has a syndrome or a particular kind of heart defect, a national support group representing those conditions should be able to help you. Make sure that you have a copy of the request in writing, and keep a note of any conversations during the assessment process.

The local authority must write within 16 weeks to tell you whether or not an EHC Plan is going to be made and the reasons for their decision. You will be told how to appeal if the decision is not to provide it.

If an EHC Plan is going ahead, you should be sent a draft and you will have 15 days to put your views forward. Look to see if all potential concerns regarding your child's needs have been properly dealt with, and you will want to look particularly at which school or educational place is named in the Plan for your child. You can ask to meet with the LA and the people who gave advice.

Home education
What about educating your child at home? Under the law in all parts of the UK as a parent you must ensure your child receives an education, whether in a school or at home or travelling abroad ..... it is your decision.

Reasons that parents of children with heart conditions have given include physical problems with getting a child to school, fitting the child's school's requirements around their medical appointments and treatments, having to use a different school for siblings and problems of arrangements.

Some parents will want to home school from the start, because they are positive about the educational experience they can give their child, unfettered by educational institutions, national curriculum, tests and schedules. If this applies to your family, let your local authority know that your child will not be taking up a school place (you don't have to do this, but there may be anxiety about what has happened to him or her if you don't).

In other cases a child may have attended a school, but has struggled to adapt, and may be lonely and unhappy, or is just not progressing in the way the family had hoped. When a child is taken out of a state school in England or Wales, the head teacher will notify the local authority and in Scotland parents have to let the local authority know. BUT if your child attends a special school you will need to deregister him or her. Home education must be suitable to the child's age, ability, aptitude and special educational needs - if your child has an Education Health and Care Plan you may want to ask the local authority for help in fulfilling those parts of it normally arranged through a school.

Your local authority will in all probability ask to visit you to look at the educational provision your children are enjoying – this is a request not a demand.

Going to school
By the time your child starts school you should have a good idea as to whether he or she is going to (or just possibly might) need extra help.

As parent of a child with a medical condition you will want to check the school's policy on how they will support your child when and if necessary. School can provide you with their policy of care for children with medical problems, including dealing with periods of absence, how they will train staff to administer medications needed at school, how they will offer opportunities to participate and so on. You can ask the local authority to assess your child for an EHC Plan at this stage. For children with medical conditions the school can draw up an individual health care plan, and your input will be important, especially for the younger child who may need frequent toileting because of diuretics, or the child who may be in danger of uncontrolled bleeding because of being on an anticoagulant, for example. Ask other parents in your support group about plans they have been involved with. Putting your child's Named Nurse in touch with the school may be a good way forward if you are having difficulties – and many of us do!

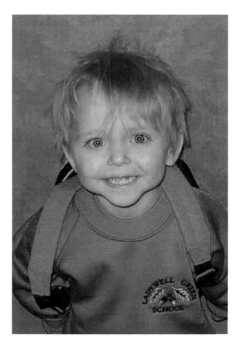

Unable to attend

There is a minimum national standard for educating children who are unable to attend school because of their medical needs. You should ask the school where this is recorded and how your child will be affected by absence. Often absence is for a period each day, when children become too fatigued to deal with full school hours. The guidance for schools says 'any period' of absence, not just those periods of several days or weeks when a child is hospitalised or at home with a long illness. Unfortunately not all schools act on the guidance so you may need to apply some pressure to make sure your child does not miss out.

Educational psychology services

Your child may be referred to the educational psychologist because of learning difficulties or behavioural, social and emotional problems.

There may be an assessment of your child in school – this can involve observing how your child interacts with others, discussion with you and your child separately, and psychometric testing. The educational psychologist's report may form part of your child's assessment for an Education Health Care plan, or support changes to it. Although schools tend to ask for a referral to the educational psychologist, as a parent you can ask your local authority directly if you have concerns about your child. It is a good idea to try to involve the school with your request, or get the support of your GP.

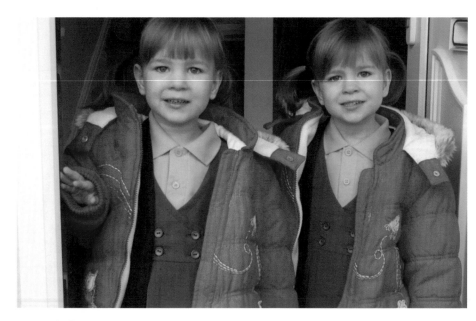

More information and support

Information here mainly relates to England – and is similar throughout the UK but there are some differences in Northern Ireland, Scotland, and Wales. Citizen Advice Bureau has websites for all four countries. Relevant help for your situation can also be found on the websites and facebook pages of many support groups – see **Chapter 13 Sources of help and support**.

National Portage Service
t: 0121 244 1807
w: www.portage.org.uk

Carers UK
t: 0808 808 7777
As a parent with a disabled child you are recognised in law as a carer, and are entitled to support from Carers UK

Health Conditions in School Alliance
w: http://medicalconditionsatschool.org.uk
Offers a number of drafts for the documentation you may want, such as policy statement and care plans.

Family and Childcare Trust
e: info@familyandchildcaretrust.org
w: www.familyandchildcaretrust.org
The Trust promotes high quality and affordable day care.

Contact a Family
t: 0808 808 3555
Detailed information and advice on different types of childcare specifically for children with disabilities and how to access it

Ofsted (England)
w: www.ofsted.gov.uk
Latest local schools and childcare facilities inspection, and registered nannies reports

Northern Ireland: Education Training Inspectorate
t: 028 9127 9726
e: inspectionservices@deni.gov.uk
w: www.etini.gov.uk

Scottish Care Inspectorate
t: 0845 600 9527
e: enquiries@careinspectorate.com
w: www.careinspectorate.com

Welsh Inspectorate for Education and Training
t: 029 2044 6446
e: enquiries@estyn.gov.uk
w: www.estyn.gov.uk

Home Education Advisory Service
t: 01707 371854
e: enquiries@heas.org.uk
w: www.heas.org.uk
For an overview of home schooling. Your local authority and local library can provide details of home schooling support, groups, charities and so on

NB
Special educational needs (SEN) are factors which prevent a child from learning in the same way as other children. In Scotland, the term "additional support needs" (ASN) is used and includes factors affecting a child's learning such as bullying, bereavement, family being in care or being a teenage parent.

The systems in Wales and Northern Ireland are broadly similar to that in England, although they both have their own codes of practice.

Most children with severe heart defects will have times when they are critically ill and their life is in the balance. Although the majority of families will experience the happiness of seeing their child recover, sadly some children die.

As a parent you may find that your ability to support a bereaved family can be impaired by increased fears for your own heart child, or maybe as a member of the health team who has struggled to sustain a child's life, you may be dealing with a sense of failure.

This chapter outlines a little of the issues and experiences of grief or loss which may be helpful to those who are close to bereaved families and can offer support through these hardest of times.

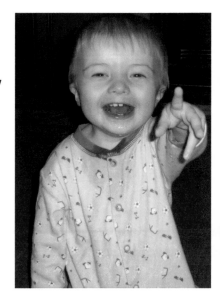

Knowing the child is dying

If it is known that the child is dying, there may be time to talk openly and honestly with the parents about expectations and fears, discuss any options and choices that might be possible. These could be about where the child should be cared for – at home, in hospital, or perhaps in a hospice – or what treatment alternatives are available, or what financial help may be needed, for example.

If there is time, you may want to help prepare other members of the family; especially younger children who may be helped by services such as those provided by pastoral care, from school, children's hospice, local hospital or the children's community nursing team. You may be able to look after a brother or sister regularly, so that when parents are preoccupied with impending bereavement, you are a trusted face.

When a child dies at home

The expected death

Even when the child is not expected to survive, death may still come as a huge shock, which prevents parents from being able to think things through as they normally would. So it may be best to make decisions beforehand, such as whether they want a funeral director or to keep the child's body at home and arrange the funeral themselves.

The unexpected death

The shock of an unexpected death is intensified for the family when they discover that it is being regarded as a sudden death – and that they have to deal with the enquiries of the police, coroner's officer and social care team.

Support for such families will mean being sensitive to the distress and anger this can cause, and understanding that the question of why the child has died is insignificant compared with the fact of the loss to the family.

When a child dies in hospital

Although parents may suspect that their child is dying, they may be afraid to ask and have their fears confirmed. Hospital staff tend to focus on the positive and may avoid voicing concerns that a child is deteriorating.

It is best for both staff and parents to face honestly the probable outcomes, trying to anticipate any choices that may need to be made in both treatment and end of life care plans. To remain trustworthy, friends will need to support parents without offering false hope or comfort, or undermining justifiable fears.

Parents need to know that they have done everything possible to prevent this death –they will re-examine every second leading up to it minutely. They will look for any of their actions which could have delayed treatment, or times when they were not at the bedside, or when they were unable to communicate with their child. Hospital staff are in a good position to help parents through this process, and protect them from unnecessary self-accusation and blame. Friends, too, should be able to listen to repeated accounts with kindliness and patience.

Immediately after the child's death in hospital

Staff will try to ensure that the family have as much time as they need to spend with the child, to cuddle, to hold, and to begin to say goodbye. They should be offered the opportunity to have photographs taken, to take a lock of hair, and have hand or foot prints, perhaps to add to a memory box. The appropriate hospital chaplain can be contacted day or night, or the family might prefer for someone from their own community to come to support them.

Every effort will be made to accommodate any particular faith rituals that they wish to be carried out. If the child does not require a post-mortem and the medical staff are able to complete the certificate of death, the child can be collected by the funeral director and taken to their Chapel of Rest, to his or her own home or to the local children's hospice if the family is known to them.

The family can transport the child themselves, as long as they have a suitable car, and a person who is able to drive safely in this situation. The hospital will need to provide a letter of authority to do this, as well as the death certificate.

If a post-mortem is needed, after the family leaves, the child will be taken to the mortuary. Ward staff will arrange for members of the family to see the child again in the mortuary viewing room whilst he or she remains in the hospital. The family may want to bring favourite clothing for the child during this time, or later to give to the funeral director.

When a child dies in a children's hospice

The expertise of staff at a children's hospice will enable the family to be supported in an environment that is more homely than hospital. All children's hospices have facilities to care for the whole family as well as the dying child and to continue this care after death until the family are ready to go home - often this is on the day of the funeral. Those helping to arrange the funeral can visit at the hospice, and funeral directors can bring a chosen casket or coffin to the cooled room where the child is being cared for.

Registering the death

The child's death has to be registered by the registrar, either in the area of the hospital or hospice or your home where the child died. This has to be done within five days.If the coroner has been involved, because of sudden death or circumstances that may require investigating, registering the death may have to be delayed. The coroner's officer will advise about this

Post mortems

The coroner can require a post mortem in order to obtain more information about the cause of death. Parents will have support and advice from the coroner's officer at this time and be kept in contact with what is happening. If the hospital doctor wants a post mortem carried out, to increase medical knowledge for the benefit of other children with a similar condition, he or she will have to ask permission and discuss the procedure with the parents, explain what is involved and ask for their written consent. Explicit permission is required for retention of any organ or tissue for any purpose - this will be fully explained to the parents.

Parents will have the opportunity to discuss the results of the hospital post mortem, once the report is prepared, and may want to see a copy. This should be discussed with them, as the terminology is, of necessity, clinical and requires some explanation. The Coroner will arrange for discussion of any post mortem results obtained under his or her authority. If there has been police involvement because of sudden death circumstances then this process can be quite lengthy.

Organ or tissue donation

Facing the tragedy of a child's death is sometimes helped by the knowledge that the gift of an organ or some tissue may help another. It is important that medical staff give families an opportunity to consider this if at all possible. If the child is in intensive care it is possible that organs as well as other tissue can be donated. Organ donation will only be considered where death is inevitable, and will never occur without the consent of the family. The transplant coordinator will be contacted on their behalf if they wish. Even if a child dies at home or in a local hospital or hospice, tissue such as corneas, skin, bone or heart valves, can be donated up to twenty-four hours after the death.

This is unlikely to be an issue that a friend will raise, but one where sensitive and informed support can be helpful.

Grief and loss

Only parents who have experienced the death of a child can fully understand the impact this brings. For some parents the feelings of bereavement will have been under the surface since their child's diagnosis. The reality of this loss comes to a peak at the death of a child, and then comes the slow ongoing process of learning to live with this permanent change. For others, having experienced the first days of bereavement, realisation that this is a permanent state comes later. There is so much to do at first, and then the terrible vacuum - so try to continue support beyond those first weeks and months.

The intense rollercoaster of emotions that grief brings can be quite unpredictable, leading to a feeling of loss of control and helplessness. The death of a child is out of the natural order of things; it feels like something that shouldn't happen. It may also be the first time a family has experienced the death of someone close, bringing a range of feelings for grandparents and brothers and sisters, as well as parents.

Each family, and each individual, will have their own way of expressing emotions and their own cultural and spiritual background to influence reactions. It is important to acknowledge that everyone is unique and that there is no 'right' or 'wrong' way to grieve. Similarly timescales can be very different for people, even within the same family.

Relationships

Having said that each one is different it is important to recognise that the support required will be individual also. Couples not unusually deal with their feelings differently and find it too painful to be of help to each other, but if you are a friend, or trusted professional, you may be of help.

Often death brings a sense of isolation, embarrassment and the 'not knowing what to say' leading to friends and colleagues avoiding the bereaved. You may find that parents welcome the companionship of a friend who will be comfortable sitting in a silence they cannot fill. A listening supporter, who can be totally nonjudgemental, allowing parents to talk about whatever they wish regarding the death of their child, is a precious resource.

The following list, drawn from an original by The Compassionate Friends, has some helpful suggestions on how you might offer support to grieving parents:

- Do express your sadness for their loss and encourage them to share with you whatever they wish, acknowledging their pain.
- Do show patience, understand their need to talk and tell their story as often as they want. This patience can be reflected onto the parents who require time and should not expect too much of themselves.
- Do talk about their child, giving positive reassurances about all their experiences, remembering happy times.
- Do give siblings some special time and attention, they are grieving too.
- Do offer practical help, the offer of a meal, doing the washing, taking other children to school etc.
- Don't avoid parents because you are uncomfortable.
- Don't talk about your own feelings: it is their child that has died and their loss you are trying to support.
- Don't try to say anything positive about the death, you cannot make it better.
- Don't reinforce any feelings of doubt or guilt; just listen to what is being said at the moment.
- Don't worry about getting it right. Being there is the most important gesture of care.

Follow up

Whether the child died in hospital, at home, or in a children's hospice, a bereaved parent should be invited by the child's lead consultant to talk over what happened. Some parents welcome this, but some may find a return visit to the hospital impossible to deal with, ask for a meeting to be arranged somewhere convenient to the consultant but off the premises.

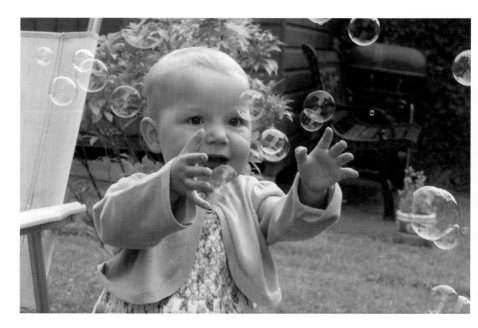

A parent may want to take a friend who can ask questions for them, or note the answers should they become distressed. If you are asked to accompany a parent be aware that they may find it too difficult to carry on. Make sure that they ask for a break in the meeting, or ask for it to be continued at a later date if this is the case.

Make sure you know who to contact and who will be able to offer help. Many of the heart organisations, such as Heartline, offer support for bereaved members, and there are many voluntary groups offering support to families, if they would like it. (There is a list at the end of this chapter).

How long the members of the family will require support will vary for each individual. Parents sometimes feel they are being disloyal to the child who died when other aspects of their lives are returning to take up some of their time. Of course, the child who has died will always remain part of the family, will never be forgotten or replaced, but learning to live without that child is essential for well being.

As a friend, assuring the family that the child is held in your memory, can help them progress towards that well being.

Capturing memories

If the funeral has not met all the family's needs, there is no reason why they should not hold a service or celebration of the child's life a little later, inviting friends and relations to contribute poems, music and stories that remind them of the child.

Every special moment is one to treasure once a child has died. It can be very helpful to gather mementoes and create a memory box or book: photographs, drawings, items the child has made themselves- all can be stored along with handprints, footprints, a lock of hair, favourite toys and books and clothing.

Expressing feelings in writing can allow for thought to flow in a way that the spoken word may not achieve. The whole family can be involved with this and enjoy reflecting on memorable events.

'Grief is not about forgetting the person who has died, but about finding ways to remember them and taking their memory forward with you in life' The Child Bereavement Charity.

There are many useful books and websites that can help with various aspects of caring for a dying child and with bereavement, as well as several organisations which can be contacted. Some of these are given here:

Child Bereavement UK
t: 0800 0288840
w: www.childbereavementuk.org

The Compassionate Friends
t: 0345 123 2304 (Northern Ireland 02887788016)
w: www.tcf.org.uk

Child Death Helpline
t: 0800 282986 (mobile 08088006019)
w: www.childdeathhelpline.org.uk

SANDS Stillbirth and Neonatal Death Society
t: 020 7436 5881
w: www.uk-sands.org

Together for Short Lives
t: 0808 8088 100
w: www.togetherforshortlives.org.uk

Organ Donation
t: 0300 123 2323
w: www.organdonation.nhs.uk

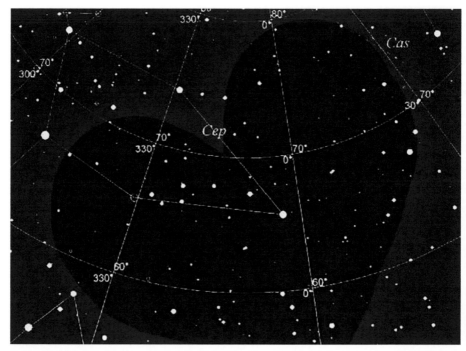

If you reach towards the sky, with Polaris, the North Star, at the heel of your hand and your fingers spread, you will be covering the area of the Heart of Stars, where Heartline families can remember their children.

13. Sources of help and support

There is a huge amount of information and support out there, in the form of books, websites, fact sheets, NHS and local authority, support group and other information. Most of it is interesting and helpful and some of it is misleading.

Searching the web – when looking for information, and particularly medical information, check the source – who wrote it and where did the writer get their information. Check the date it was written – we live in fast moving times and what was significant and important 10 years ago may be irrelevant today. If there is anything that is at odds with advice you have had from your child's cardiologist – don't take it until you have queried it with the doctor.

American sites are often very informative, but remember that health services vary from hospital to hospital and from state to state, and private medicine sites may also offer visions of care which are not possible within the NHS.

The list on the following pages was up-to-date when we went to print, and concentrates on only the most relevant areas for families with heart children.

Support groups

Barth Syndrome Trust (BST)
t: 01794 518785
e: info@barthsyndrome.org.uk
w: www.barthsyndrome.org.uk

Saving lives through education, advances in treatment and finding a cure for Barth Syndrome.

The Brompton Fountain
t: 03300229291
e: admin@thebromptonfountain.org.uk
w: www.thebromptonfountain.org.uk

The Brompton Fountain is a parent support for families whose children are being treated for cardiac and respiratory conditions at the Royal Brompton and Harefield NHS Trust.

Cardiac Risk in the Young – also known as CRY
t: 01737 363222
e: cry@c-r-y.org.uk
w: www.c-r-y.org.uk

CRY supports young people diagnosed with potentially lifethreatening cardiac conditions and offers bereavement support to families affected by sudden cardiac death in the young. CRY promotes and develops heart screening programmes and funds medical research.

Cardiomyopathy UK
t: 0800 0181 024
e: info@cardiomyopathy.org
w: www.cardiomyopathy.org

We help people with cardiomyopathy and their families find all the information they need to manage the condition. We are here to support from diagnosis to receiving specialist care and undergoing family genetic testing.

Children's Heart Association
t: 01706 221988
e: information@heartchild.info
w: www.heartchild.info

We are the families and friends of children with congenital heart disorders. The Children's Heart Association has four main aims: to give support and understanding to parents and families, to improve facilities for children at heart units, to maintain standards of improvement as new techniques develop, and to raise funds to help purchase specialised equipment.

Children's Heart Federation
t: 08088085000
w: www.chfed.org.uk

CHF is a federation of support groups in the UK and Ireland for families with (or expecting) a child with a heart condition.

A large number of fact sheets can be downloaded from the website or ordered by telephone. These cover many of the heart conditions that children are born with or acquire, and related issues for families with heart children.

Children's Heart Unit Fund
t: 01912813166
e: info@chuf.org.uk
w: www.chuf.org.uk

The Children's Heart Unit at the Freeman Hospital Newcastle is just one of two in the UK that has the facilities and skills to offer pediatric transplant and bridge to transplant operations. As a result, the Unit treats critically ill babies and children from across the UK. All CHUF's work goes towards raising funds and awareness to maintain and improve that support.

Down's Heart Group
t: 0300 102 1644
e: info@dhg.org.uk
w: www.dhg.org.uk

DHG welcomes anyone with an interest in heart conditions associated with Down's Syndrome. It offers a helpline, personalised info pack, parent matching, conferences, newsletters and website.

Evelina Children's Heart Organisation (ECHO)
t: 07715208077
e: admin@echo.org.uk
w: www.echo-evelina.org.uk

ECHO is a support group for parents and families of children suffering from heart disease who are treated at the London Evelina Children's Hospital within Guy's and St Thomas' Trust.

Heartbeat - Northern Ireland
t: 0289031228
e: info@childrensheartbeattrust.org
w: www.childrensheartbeattrust.org

Heartbeat - NI provides emotional and practical support to families and financial support to Clark Clinic at Royal Belfast Hospital for Sick Children.

Heart Children Ireland
t: Lo Call 1850 217017 (within Republic of Ireland)
From the UK 00353 1 8740990
e: heartchildren@eircom.net
w: www.heartchildren.ie

Membership is open to parents and families of children with a congenital heart disorder. Services include a quarterly magazine, professional counselling service, social events where parents can meet, annual conference, and annual bereaved service.

Heartline Families
t: 03300 224466
e: admin@Heartline.org.uk
w: www.Heartline.org.uk

Heartline supports children with heart disorders and their families, whatever the condition, wherever it is treated and has a national membership of nearly 3000 throughout the UK. We publish this book - **Heart Children** - which is provided free to our members, provide help and advice through booklets, newsletters, magazine and social media. Families can benefit from free wetsuits for a heart child, caravan holidays and short activity breaks.

Heart Link
t: 0500 382152
e: info@heartlink-glenfield.org.uk
w: www.heartlink-glenfield.org.uk

Membership is open to heart children treated at Glenfield Hospital and their families. Heart Link offers a parental support group and fundraising to support Glenfield Hospital.

Lagan's Foundation
t: 07486 313296
w: www.lagans.org.uk

Lagan's Foundation offers home respite and support services for young children with heart defects or feeding issues, providing parents with a volunteer for a minimum of two hours a week.

Little Hearts Matter
t: 0121 455 8982
e: info@lhm.org.uk
w: www.lhm.org.uk

Offers support and information to children, and their families, diagnosed with a single ventricle heart condition where a Fontan procedure is the planned treatment. The charity also works to raise the profile of the needs of these children within political, educational and social arenas.

Max Appeal!
t: 0300 999 2211
e: info@maxappeal.org.uk
w: www.maxappeal.org.uk

Membership is for people whose family is affected by DiGeorge syndrome, VCFS and 22q11.2 deletion. Services are a newsletter, helpline, meetings both national and local, website, information and parent contact.

Patches
t: 07960868843
e: patches.info@ymail.com
w: http://patchesheartgroup.webs.com

Patches supports children with congenital and acquired heart conditions in the community, including those whose children have complex needs due to genetic conditions or syndromes, offering friendly parent-to-parent information and signposting 24/7 on helpline and facebook family support group.

The Scottish Association for Children with Heart Disorders
e: secretary@youngheart.info
w: www.youngheart.info

The Scottish Association for Children with Heart Disorders offers support and understanding in everyday care and welfare to parents and families of children with heart disorders and seek to improve facilities for children and young adults at heart units and in hospitals throughout Scotland. There are a number of local area branches and a young adults' group.

Somerville Foundation
t: 0800 854759
e: helpline@thesf.org.uk
w: www.thesf.org.uk

The Somerville Foundation works with young people and adults born with a heart condition (congenital) providing practical and emotional support and enabling them to take control of their lives and manage their own heart condition.

Tiny Tickers
e: info@TinyTickers.org
w: www.TinyTickers.org

We are concerned with improving the detection of congenital heart disease before birth, by raising awareness and training healthcare professionals in NHS hospitals in the UK.

Young Hearts
e: support@younghearts.org.uk
w: www.younghearts.org.uk

Young Hearts supports families with children with heart conditions in the six counties served by the Oxford University NHS Trust: Oxfordshire, Gloucestershire, Wiltshire, Berkshire, Buckinghamshire and Northants. Our main aims are to raise funds, provide factual information and support to parents who are facing what perhaps we faced when our own children were going through difficulties.

We also represent parents and children's views to all interested parties – the Oxford University Hospitals Trust, clinicians and administrators in the NHS, local MPs and the media.

Other help and support organisations

Bliss – The Premature Baby Charity
t: 0500 6181340
e: ask@bliss.org.uk
w: www.bliss.org.uk

Bliss offers parents and families of preterm or sick babies cover and support from birth to five years, helpline, message board, enquiries email, publications, and Shared Experience register. Bliss has local branches providing up to date information and support to families.

British Heart Foundation
t: 03003303311
w: www.bhf.org.uk

BHF has a number of resources for parents and children including a DVD: 'Little Hearts, Big Questions - children with congenital heart disease' - for families of newly-diagnosed children, 'Sammy's Heart Operation' - a book for children 6-11 preparing for heart surgery, and meet@teenheart: website resources for young people from diagnosis to leaving home.

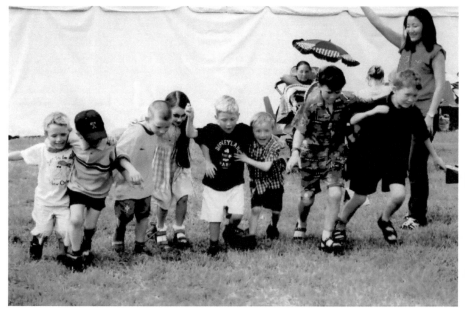

Joining a support group can provide reassurance for patients – and is great fun for the children!

Contact a Family
t: 0808 808 3555
e: info@cafamily.org.uk
w: www.cafamily.org.uk

Contact a Family provides advice, information and support to parents of all disabled children - no matter what their health condition – and offer a parent linking service at www.makingcontact.org.

A freephone helpline offers advice on welfare rights, community care issues, education needs and a listening ear with access to interpreters. There are a number of local, regional and national offices plus volunteer family workers around the UK.

Marfan Association UK
t: 01252 810472
e: contactus@marfan-association.org.uk
w: www.marfan-association.org.uk

Membership is open to anyone with an interest in Marfan syndrome or affected by Marfan syndrome. The Association offers support, education, research nationally, and collaborating internationally.

Together for Short Lives
t: 08088088100
w: www.togetherforshortlives.org.uk

Together for Short Lives is for all children with life-threatening and life-limiting conditions and all those who support, love and care for them. We support families, professionals and services, including children's hospices.

Twins and Multiple Births Association
t: 0800 138 0509
w: www.tamba.org.uk

Tamba has advice and information about what to expect while you are pregnant. If you are already a parent to twins or more, we have lots of useful information for you too, from breast feeding advice to information about schooling.

Unique
t: 01883723356
e: info@rarechromo.org
w: www.rarechromo.co.uk

Unique is a source of information and support to families and individuals affected by any rare chromosome disorder and to the professionals who work with them.

Waving Not Drowning
t: 03000120312
e: advice@working families.org.uk

The Waving Not Drowning Campaign is for parents of disabled children who want to combine paid work with their caring responsibilites. There is a dedicated helpline for queries about work and the provision of suitable affordable childcare, increased availability of flexible working and paid time off to accompany children to appointments.

Websites

There are literally hundreds of websites which may be helpful, but the most useful for finding information on children's heart matters will probably be Children's Heart Federation, or a support group for the kind of disability your child may have, and Contact a Family for up-to-date and wide-ranging information.

Your support group may have a site which provides details of your child's heart hospital environs – where to shop, eat, and relax.

For information provided by the National Institute for Cardiovascular Research (NICOR) see their Congenital Heart Disease Audit website. This gives a lot of detail about the different units, including the outcomes of the surgeries and catheter procedures carried out there.

Healthtalkonline is a site that provides not just lots of information about a subject, but parent and patient experience as well, in the form of interviews, video clips: see www.healthtalkonline.org/heart_disease/Congenital_Heart_Disease

People

Talk to your librarian and your child's teacher, about what books and DVDs are available to help your child and brothers and sisters. They are also a valuable source of advice as to what is going on in your local area.

Index

Look for words and abbreviations which are not covered here in the Terms section which follows.

Carbon Dioxide	7, 10, 24
Cardiac catheter	21, 82, 99
Cardiac Liaison Nurse (CLN)	65, 99
Cardiomyopathy	15, 37, 42, 82
Cardiorespiratory	71
Cardioversion	54
Carer's Allowance	127, 128
Catheter	12, 19, 21, 22, 26, 27, 29, 31, 35-38, 40, 41, 43, 45, 47-49, 51-54, 56, 57, 60, 61, 63, 67-75, 77-80, 82, 88, 93, 99, 102, 104, 154
Catheter Lab Technician	99
Central Venous Catheter	88
Chaplain	99, 139
Charge Nurse	98, 99, 101
Chest pain	18
Chest tubes	111
Chest x-ray	23, 46, 108
Child Bereavement Charity	143
Child Death Helpline	144
Childminder	132, 133
Children's Heart Federation (CHF)	2, 13, 39, 95, 129, 146, 152
Child Tax Credits	113, 127
Chloride	66
Chlorothiazide	66
Chyle	88
Chylothorax	80
Circulation	7, 10, 11, 13, 16-18, 26, 28, 41, 43, 44, 45, 47-50, 56, 57, 69, 72, 75, 79, 80, 88, 108
Citizens Advice Bureau (CAB)	128
Closed heart surgery	69, 70
Clubbing	16
Coarctation of the Aorta	36, 72
Coil	46, 72, 80
Collaterals	76
Community Health Council	96
Community Team	113
Compassionate Friends, The	141, 144
Competitive sport	30
Complaints procedure	98
Complete Atrio-Ventricular Septal Defect (CAVSD)	32
Complete Heart Block	32, 34, 35

Donor valve	41
Double Inlet Left Ventricle (DILV)	38
Double Inlet Right Ventricle (DIRV)	38
Double Inlet Ventricle	38
Down's Syndrome	147
Drain	8, 27, 71, 80, 81, 109, 112
Drip	21, 87, 109
Drugs	65-67, 76, 87-89, 98, 99, 109
Duct	8, 10, 26, 41-43, 45-48, 50, 58, 72, 80, 81
Ductus Arteriosus	11, 44, 45, 47, 49, 50, 55, 56, 72, 75

E

Early Years Foundation Stage Framework (EYFS)	132
Ebstein's Anomaly	39
ECG Technician	100
Echocardiogram	30, 46, 116
Echocardiography	22
Education	133-135, 137, 145, 151
Education Health Care (EHC) Plan	133
Educational Psychologist	135
Electrocardiogram	20, 44
Electrophysiological tests	71
Embryo	10
Employment	26, 98, 124, 129, 130
Enalapril	67
Endocarditis	15, 116, 117
Epilepsy	52
Event Recorder	20
Exercise Tolerance	17, 25
Exertion	118, 119
Expressed milk	63
Extra-Cardiac Fontan	74
Extra Corporeal Membrane Oxygenation (ECMO)	71

F

Facemask	109
Failure to Thrive	17, 63
Fainting	17, 18, 20, 30, 42
Faith rituals	139
Fallot's Tetralogy (FT, TOF)	26, 40, 66, 73
Family Information Service	132

Terms

This list of terms explains some of the words, phrases and abbreviations you may hear but which are not necessarily explained in this book. If you are unsure about the meaning of anything, ask the person who wrote it, your GP or Named Nurse. Can't find it here? Look in the Index.

A

Abscess – a localised collection of infected liquid called pus
Acidosis – loss of the normal balance of body chemistry resulting from poor heart action and poor blood supply to parts of the body
Anaemia – reduction in the red blood cell count
Anaesthesia – the state produced by an anaesthetic
Anaesthetic – a chemical that produces loss of consciousness
Analgesic – a chemical substance that produces freedom from pain
Aneurysm – a ballooning of the wall of a blood vessel or of the heart
Angiography – a procedure to see blood vessels using x-ray by first injecting a dye
Angioplasty – stretching of a narrow artery by a balloon catheter
Anomalous – wrong
Anomaly – something wrong
Aortic arch – topmost part of the aorta from which the head, neck and arm arteries arise
ARP – anticipated recovery pathway
Artery – a blood vessel that carries blood away from the heart
Ascites – fluid in the abdomen
Asystole – stoppage of heart action
Atheroma – damage to the lining of arteries producing narrowing and reduction of blood flow onto which clots may form
Atresia – blocked/missing/never formed
Autopsy – examination of the body after death
Autograft – using the body's own tissue

B

Banding – an artificial narrowing of the lung artery with a 'band' or string to reduce blood flow
Bifurcation – division into two
Bicuspid – having two cusps
Biopsy – removal of a small piece of tissue
Blalock-Taussig shunt – operation to join left or right subclavian artery to pulmonary artery
Blood pressure – the pressure of blood within the vessels
BNO – Bowels not opened

BO – Bowels opened **BP** – Blood pressure
Bronchomalacia – softening of the cartilage supporting the two bronchi
Bronchus (plural is bronchi) – main airway to each lung
Bundle of His – part of the system of conducting nerves in the heart

C

Caesarian – a surgical operation to removed the baby from the uterus through the wall of the abdomen
Capillaries – very fine blood vessels through whose walls food, oxygen, waste products, carbon dioxide are filtered to and from the body tissues
Carbon dioxide – waste gas produced as a by-product of body activity
Cardiac – to do with the heart
Cardiac output – the amount of blood pumped by the heart per minute
Cardiomyopathy – disease of the heart muscle
Cardioplegia – a chemical solution used to protect heart muscle during open heart surgery
Cardiopulmonary bypass – a pump and an oxygenator to maintain blood supply to the body while the heart's action is stopped
Cardioversion – shocking a heart into a normal rhythm
Cholesterol – a fatty chemical found particularly in animal fat
Chordae tendonae – fibrous cords that support the mitral and tricuspid valves
Chorea – spontaneous abnormal purposeless movements
Chromosomes – in every cell, DNA bonded to proteins that carry genes Chronotrope – to increase heart rate
Circulation – the system of heart, veins and arteries for getting oxygen and nutrients in the blood to the organs, and carrying deoxygenated blood back
Chyle – a fluid containing a lot of fat within the lymphatic system
Clinical governance – regular review by hospital clinicians and managers to maintain ethical standards
Clubbing – rounded swelling of the ends of the fingers or toes
Coil – a device used for blocking blood vessels
Collaterals – natural additional blood vessels to help overcome a blockage
Conducting – carrying an electrical signal
Conduit – artificial tube Congenital – present at birth
Congenital Heart Disease, Condition, Defect - abnormality of the heart present at birth
Congestion – too much fluid in a part of the body
Consolidation – part of lungs becoming airless Convulsion – a fit
Coronary arteries – the blood supply to the heart muscle
Coroner – an official who inquires into unnatural death eg sudden, unexpected or those related to procedures or operations
Corrective – to return the circulation to normal
CPAP – constant positive airway pressure, a way of keeping small airspaces open
Cyanosis – blue colouration of skin and lips due to lower amount of oxygen in the capillaries

D

Defibrillator – a machine using electrical shock to treat abnormalities of heart rhythm
Descending aorta – the aorta beyond the aortic arch
Dialysis – a method of washing out waste products
Diaphragm – muscle of breathing that separates the chest from the abdomen
Diastole – resting phase of heart action
Diastolic blood pressure – the lower of the blood pressure readings, produced as the heart relaxes
Doppler – the use of sound waves to assess speed and direction of blood flow
Drain – a tube used to move fluid or air from the body
Drip – a means of getting food and drugs into a vein
Duct – a tube carrying fluid or blood
Ductus arteriosus – a blood vessel part of the embryo's circulation, carrying blood from the pulmonary artery to the aorta Should close shortly after birth
Dysphagia – difficulty with swallowing
Dyspnoea – breathlessness

E

ECG – electrocardiogram: recording of the electrical activity of the heart
Echocardiogram – a picture of the heart and blood vessels using reflected high frequency sound waves
ECMO – Extra Corporeal Membrane Oxygenation: a heart lung machine – which may be used to rest the heart and lungs
-ectomy – removal
EEG - electro-encephalogram – recording electrical activity of the brain
EF - Ejection Fraction – percentage of blood pumped from the ventricle
Electrocardiogram – recording of the electrical activity of the heart
Electrodes – fine wires that carry electrical activity from or into the heart
Embolus – an abnormal substance within the blood stream such as clot or air
Embryo – the developing baby within the womb
Endocarditis – inflammation of the endocardium
Endocardium – smooth lining on the inside of the heart and its valves

F

Failure – inability of the organ to cope with demands
Failure to thrive – poor or no weight gain
Fainting – temporary loss of consciousness
Familial – runs in families
Femoral – related to the leg
Fetal – of the fetus – the baby before birth
Fibrillation – disorganised heart contractions
Flutter – abnormally fast regular beating usually of the atrium
Fetus – sometime spelt 'foetus' – developing baby within the womb

G

Gastrostomy – a hole created so that food can be fed directly into the stomach
Gene – an inherited characteristic, a part of a chromosome

H

Haematoma – a localised collection of blood outside a vessel
Haemoglobin – the chemical carried in red cells that carries oxygen, carbon dioxide and gives colour to the blood
Haemolysis – destruction of red cells
Haemoptysis – blood coughed up from lungs
Haemorrhage – a leak of blood from blood vessels
Hb – haemoglobin
Heart block – disturbance in heart rhythm so that the ventricles beat more slowly then the atriums, described as first degree, second degree or complete
Heart-lung machine, Heart-lung bypass machine – oxygenates and pumps blood around the body while heart operations are carried out
Heterograft – (also called Xenograft) – using a tissue from another species
Homograft (also called allograft) – using tissue from another human
Hyper – too much
Hypertension – elevated blood pressure
Hyperthermia – very high temperature Hypo – too little
Hypoplastic – underdeveloped
Hypotension – low blood pressure
Hypothermia – very low temperature

I

Idiopathic – cause unknown
Immunisation – a method of increasing patient's defence against infection
Incompetence – leaking
Infant – less than one year
Infarct – death of tissue related to blocking of the blood supply
Infective endocarditis – acquired heart disease
Infra – below
Infusion – fluid or medication given slowly into a vein
Inotrope – a drug used to increase heart muscle function
Intra – within
Intravenous infusion (IV) - giving drugs or fluids directly into a vein
Intubation – passage of a tube into the windpipe to assist with breathing
Ischaemia – reduction in organ function as a result of reduced blood supply
-itis – infection
Invasive test, invasive procedure – the skin needs to be penetrated
IVs – intravenous infusions

J

Jaundice – yellow colouring of skin and eyes as a result of liver dysfunction or red cell breakdown
Juxta – nearby

K

Keloid – a hard lumpy scar from excess fibrous tissue

L

Leucocyte – white blood cell that fights infection
Lines – intravenous and intra-arterial cannulae Lobe – part of an organ
Lymph – body fluid running in channels, drains fluid and particularly fats from the bowel back into the circulation

M

Macro – large
Mediastinum – space in the chest between the lungs, heart and great vessels
Micro – small
Monocusp – a single cusp from a donor valve
Murmur – noise produced by blood flow in the heart and vessels

N

Nasogastric – from nose to stomach
NBM – nil by mouth
Needle phobia - fear of injections
Neonate – baby in the first month of life
NG – nasogastric
NGT – nasogastric tube
NO – Nitric oxide
Node – area of specialised cell that controls the rhythm of the heart
Non-invasive test, non-invasive procedure – does not need to penetrate the skin
NPU – not passed urine
Nucleus – central part of most cells and contains the chromosomes
Nutrients – those parts of food which are used by the body for repair and growth

O

O2 – oxygen
Obs – observations
Oedema – extra fluid accumulating in the tissue
Oesophagus – gullet
OHS
Oliguria – too little urine

- ology – the study of
- ostomy – a hole
- otomy – an incision
OPD – outpatient department
Outpatients – a department of a hospital your child may visit without being admitted to the hospital
Oximeter – a machine to measure oxygen
Oxygen – part of the air that is needed by all animal cells for normal working
Oxygenator – an artificial machine that delivers oxygen into the blood

P

Pacemaker – electrical control of the speed of the heart – either natural or artificial
Paediatric – old spelling of pediatric
Palliation – a procedure to improve the patient's condition
Palpitation – an uncomfortable sensation of heart beat which may be slow, fast, irregular or regular
Parasympathetic nerves – nerves to the heart that slow heart rate
Parenteral – medicines or fluids given by injection
Paresis – paralysis
PCU – Pediatric Cardiac Unit: part of a hospital which specialises in treating children with heart conditions
PDA – Patent ductus arteriosus
Pediatric – sometimes spelt 'paediatric' – word to describe science of medical problems in children
Pediatric cardiologist – doctor specialising in children's heart conditions
Peri – nearby
Pericardium – lining bag in which the heart sits
Peritoneum – membrane lining the inside of the abdomen
Phrenic nerve – nerve that supplies the diaphragm
Physiological – functioning normally
Placenta – organ inside the uterus that supplies the developing baby with nourishment and removes waste products
Plasma – liquid part of the blood
Platelets – small particles in the blood which are important for blood clotting
Pleura – covering layer of the lungs and the inside of the chest
Pneumothorax – air outside the lung and within the chest cavity
Polycythaemia – increased number of red blood cells
Precordium – part of the chest in front of the heart
Prenatal diagnosis – finding out about the baby's condition before birth
Procedure – another word for operation or treatment or invasive test
Prognosis – an estimation of outlook for the patient's particular problem
Prophylaxis – prevention
Prosthetic – artificial
PU – passed urine
Pulmonary – of the lungs
Pulse – the arterial beat from forward blood flow produced by the heart contraction

Pulse oximeter – a device for measuring oxygen in the blood
Pus – liquid produced by infection
Pyrexia – high temperature

R

Radiograph – photograph of part of the body using x-rays
Radio-isotope – a substance uses radioactivity for diagnostic purposes
Re-entry circuit - continual electrical reactivation of part of the heart
Regurgitant – backward flow – leaking
Renal – pertaining to kidneys
Resuscitation – treatment to stimulate the heart or breathing

S

Sac – bag
Saline – salt solution usually the same strength as body fluid
Saphenous – a vein in the leg
Sats – short for oxygen saturation
Sclerosis – hardening of tissue
Scoliosis – curvature of the spine
Sedation – drugs used to reduce nervousness and increase calm, reduced level of consciousness
Semilunar – crescent shaped, relates to the aortic or pulmonary valve leaflets
Septectomy – removal of a septum
Septicaemia – an infection of the blood stream
Septostomy – a hole created in the septum
Septum – a dividing structure
Shock – severe failure of the circulation with cessation of normal body action Shunt – a natural or artificial tube used to increase blood supply to the lungs
Side effects - ways in which a medicine can affect the patient, other than the way intended
Sign – an abnormality found on examination
Sphygmomanometer – instrument for measuring blood pressure
Stenosis – narrowing in the vessel or valve
Stent – an expandable metal tube used to enlarge narrow vessels
Sternum – breast bone
Stillbirth – birth of a baby who has died
Stridor – noisy breathing
Stroke – loss of function related to blockage or bursting of blood vessel supplying part of the brain
Sub – below
Subclavian – below the clavicle
Supra – above
Suture – fine string used to sew two parts together
SVT – Supra Ventricular Tachycardia – a fast heart beat starting in the atrial chambers
Sympathetic nerve – nerves to the heart that increase the heart rate

Symptom – an indication of a medical condition
Syncope – loss of consciousness related to lack of blood flow to the brain
Syndrome – a collection of abnormalities that together produce a recognisable pattern
Systole – the period of contraction of the ventricles
Systolic blood pressure – the top of blood pressure measurement taken when the heart is contracting

T

Tachycardia – rapid heart rate
Tachypnoea – rapid breathing
Tamponade – obstruction to filling of the heart by pressure from a surrounding collection of fluid
Thoracic duct – vessel carrying lymph drainage from bowel through the chest to the subclavian vein
Thoracotomy – an operation on the chest
Threshold – lowest level of stimulus that will produce a response
Thrill – vibration that can be felt, produced by abnormal blood flow
Thrombolysis – dissolving a clot in a blood vessel with drugs
Thrombosis – clot formation
Thrombus – clot
Toxic – an illness related to a poisonous by-product usually infection
Trachea – windpipe
Tracheomalacia – softening of the cartilage that supports the windpipe
Tracheostomy – a small tube inserted through a hole in the windpipe to assist breathing

U

Umbilical – tube that connects the placenta to the developing baby before birth
Umbrella – a catheter device to block abnormal blood vessel
Unifocalisation – bringing separate vessels together

V

Vaccine – a liquid of weak or killed micro-organisms, or their proteins that that can be used to prevent diseases
VAD – ventricular assist device to support the heart
Vagus nerve – nerve supply to the body and bowel, stimulation of which slows the heart rate
Valve – structure which opens and closes to allow blood flow in one direction only
Valvoplasty – stretching of a narrow valve often with a balloon catheter
Valvotomy – cutting or stretching of a narrow valve
Vascular – relating to blood vessels
Vasodilator – a drug to open up blood vessels
Vegetation – lumpy areas on a heart valve caused by infection and blood clot
Vein (vena) – thin walled blood vessel carrying blood towards the heart

Viral – caused by a virus
Vitamin k – helps blood to clot and is suppressed by warfarin, an anticoagulant

X

Xenograft – tissue from another species
X-ray – a test using rays to see the more solid structures inside the body

Show me

You may find it helpful for your consultant to use these pages to explain your child's heart condition.

Your child's heart - diagnosis

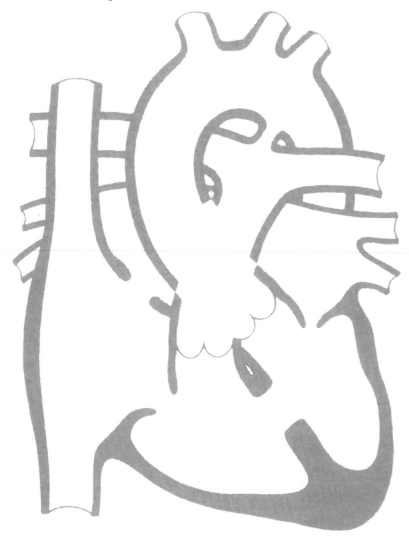

Your child's heart - after treatment

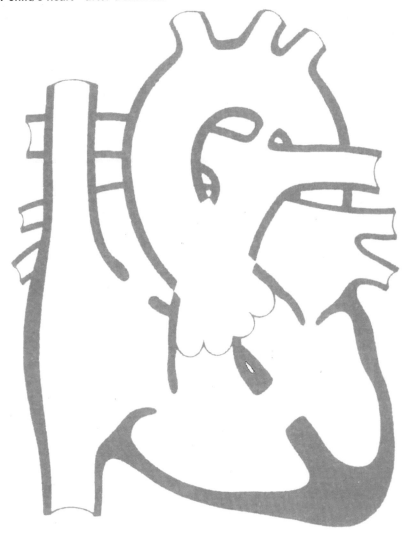